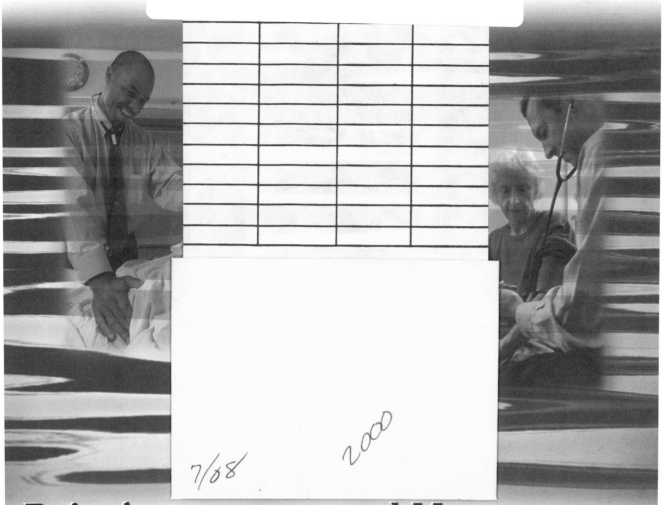

7/08

2000

Pain Assessment and Management

An Organizational Approach

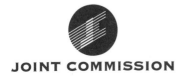

JOINT COMMISSION

Joint Commission Mission

The mission of the Joint Commission on Accreditation of Healthcare Organizations is to continuously improve the safety and quality of care provided to the public through the provision of health care accreditation and related services that support performance improvement in health care organizations.

Joint Commission educational programs and publications support, but are separate from, the accreditation activities of the Joint Commission. Attendees at Joint Commission educational programs and purchasers of Joint Commission publications receive no special consideration or treatment in, or confidential information about, the accreditation process.

Printed in the U.S.A. 5 4 3 2 1

Requests for permission to reprint or make copies of any part of this book should be addressed to:

Permissions Editor
Joint Commission on Accreditation of Healthcare Organizations
One Renaissance Boulevard
Oakbrook Terrace, IL 60181

ISBN: 0-86688-680-X

Library of Congress Catalog Number: 00-102701

For more information about the Joint Commission, please visit our Web site at www.jcaho.org.

ACKNOWLEDGMENTS

This publication is supported by an unrestricted education grant provided by Purdue Pharma L.P. (www.partnersagainstpain.com).

Pain Assessment and Management

We are indebted to our clinical and technical reviewers, including

June L. Dahl, PhD, Professor of Pharmacology, University of Wisconsin Medical School

Patricia Berry, PhD, RN, CRNH, CS, Project Coordinator, Institutionalizing Pain Management, A Project of the Robert Wood Johnson Foundation

Chapter 1:

CONTENTS

List of Figures

Chapter 1:

PAIN MANAGEMENT TODAY

Pain is the most common reason individuals seek medical attention. According to the American Pain Society (APS), 50 million Americans are partially or totally disabled by pain, and 45% of all Americans seek care for persistent pain at some point in their lives.[1] A recent study in the *New England Journal of Medicine* finds that children dying of cancer are not given adequate treatment for pain, shortness of breath, fatigue, nausea, and other symptoms.[2]

The conclusion? Pain is undertreated—despite the availability of effective pharmacologic and nonpharmacologic therapies. Why? First, according to the American Medical Association's Council on Scientific Affairs, health care professionals may have inadequate knowledge of analgesic pharmacology and pain therapy, poor pain assessment practices, and ungrounded concern about regulatory oversight.[3] They may also fear the side effects of opioid analgesics—in particular, tolerance and addiction. And they may be more focused on curing the underlying diseases than on treating pain. Second, individuals may contribute to the undertreatment problem by their reluctance to both report pain and take pain medications. Finally, too few health care systems currently make pain management a high priority.

Moreover, they may have inadequate or inappropriate provisions for reimbursement.

The Joint Commission recognizes pain as a major, yet largely avoidable, problem. To that end, it has expanded the scope of its pain management standards, which have been endorsed by the American Pain Society (APS), to cover all pain scenarios in accredited health care organizations rather than limiting the scope to end-of-life care.

This book discusses the Joint Commission's expanded requirements for pain management in hospitals; long term care organizations, including long term care pharmacies; home care organizations; ambulatory care centers; behavioral health care facilities; and health care networks. This chapter addresses the need for an organizational commitment to pain management, offers a step-by-step approach to achieving that commitment, and gives an overview of the new Joint Commission standards.

What Is Pain?

The International Association for the Study of Pain gives this definition: *Pain* is "an unpleasant sensory and emotional experience associated with actual or potential tissue damage, or described in terms of such damage or both." Pain may include a range of physical and mental sensations, such as aching, tightness, numbness, and burning. These sensations may vary in severity, persistence, source, and management. Unrelieved pain can have negative physiological and psychological effects. For example, pain interferes significantly with mobility, sleep, eating, concentration, and social interactions, causing anxiety and distress.[1] As is the case with hospitalized patients, pain in long term care residents is associated with impairments in activities of daily living and mood.[2]

Physiological effects of pain include impaired gastrointestinal and pulmonary function, nausea and dyspnea, increased metabolic rate, impaired immune response, insomnia, delayed healing, immobility-related complications, and loss of appetite. Unrelieved pain also causes anxiety, depression, fear, stress, loss of enjoyment of life, and an inability to relate to others. Physical symptoms accompanying pain include fatigue, insomnia, and weight loss. Pain also impacts family functioning, including increased social isolation and marital conflict, reduced sexual activity, and feelings of anger and resentment. Not surprisingly, anxiety and depression are associated with both the level of pain and dissatisfaction with the pain control an individual experiences.[3]

Pain can be classified as either acute or chronic. *Acute pain* is caused by an injury, illness, or surgery. It generally lasts less than six months, and usually disappears when the underlying cause has been treated or has healed. Acute pain usually responds to pain medications and other nonpharmacologic interventions. However, unrelieved acute pain may lead to chronic pain problems that result in longer hospital stays, rehospitalizations, visits to outpatient clinics and emergency departments, and increased costs.

Chronic pain exists beyond an expected time for healing, typically for six months or more. It is a persistent pain state that may be associated with a long-term incurable or intractable medical condition or disease. Approximately 9% of the U.S. adult population suffer from moderate to severe noncancer-related pain. The majority of those suffering from chronic pain have been living with their pain for over five years, on average almost six days in a typical week.[1] Determining the cause of the pain (nociceptive or neuropathic) can help the clinician select appropriate management strategies.

The Undertreatment Problem

Despite the ever-growing list of options and methods for relieving pain, pain management has shown little improvement over the past few decades. Consequently, a large percentage of hospitalized patients, regardless of why they are admitted, still experience considerable pain.[1] How large a percentage? Estimates say anywhere from 50% to 80% of patients. In one study, nearly 50% of severely ill hospitalized patients reported pain, almost 15% of whom said they had moderately or extremely severe pain at least half the time.[3] Another study reported that 50% of hospitalized patients had pain when they were interviewed, while 67% had experienced pain during the past 24 hours.[1] In a study of randomly selected hospitalized medical and surgical patients, 80% reported pain, with 45% describing it as "excruciating."[5] And according to the Institute of Medicine, a significant portion of dying persons and persons with advanced disease experience serious pain.[6] Finally, the 1992 *Clinical Practice Guideline for Acute Pain Management* of the Agency for Healthcare Research and Quality (AHRQ) suggests that routine orders for intramuscular (IM) injections of opioid "as needed" (PRN) leave more than half of postoperative patients with unrelieved pain due to undertreatment.

Hospitals are not the only settings in which individuals experience significant pain. The American Geriatrics Society suggests that between 45% and 80% of long term care residents have substantial, undertreated pain.[7] In one study, more than 70% of long term care residents reported a pain problem. When asked to describe the pain, 66% of the residents described intermittent pain, while 34% had chronic pain. Major sources of pain include the lower back, arthritis, previous fracture sites, and neuropathies.[8] One study found that approximately 40% of long term care residents with cancer experience daily pain,[9] and 25% of them do not receive analgesics.[2, 9]

What Is Pain Management?

The term *pain management* refers to a comprehensive approach to the needs of patients, residents, clients, or other individuals served who experience problems associated with acute or chronic pain. By addressing the barriers to effective pain management, a comprehensive pain management process can improve the current scenario. It usually entails an organizationwide, interdisciplinary effort, meaning that it includes medical, nursing, pharmacy, and allied health professionals whose aim is to make pain assessment and management a priority in an organization's day-to-day processes.

For patients, residents, clients, or other individuals served, an organizationwide interdisciplinary pain management initiative has these benefits: improved outcomes during service and postdischarge; increased knowledge and awareness about pain issues for both the individual served and his or her family; and increased satisfaction. Staff benefits include improved pain assessment skills, improved compliance with documentation requirements, increased knowledge of pain management issues, and greater satisfaction with the provision of care.

Barriers to Pain Management

It is true that people with pain are sometimes reluctant to report it, and some are even reluctant to take pain medications. However, even those who do report pain often do not receive appropriate treatment. Despite planned interventions from nurses to encourage physicians to address pain control, between 74% and 95% of very ill and dying hospitalized adults experience a high incidence of uncontrolled pain.[10] As noted, many health care professionals lack the knowledge and skills to manage pain effectively, and they fear the effects of treatment.[11, 12, 13, 14, 15, 16]

Lack of knowledge about analgesic pharmacology and pain therapy. Few health care professionals believe that they received adequate training in pain management in medical school or during their residency.[17, 18] As a result, they often do not prescribe opioids or nonsteroidal anti-inflammatory drugs (NSAIDs) on a regular basis, leaving patients without adequate pain relief.[19] Moreover, health care professionals are rarely aware if they have prescribed insufficient analgesic treatment.

Health care professionals may also be unaware of current best medicating practices. If they are following traditional patterns of professional practice, they may not assess and document pain. Other outdated clinical practices include undermining or failing to accept the individual's self-report of pain, prescribing IM analgesics on a PRN basis, and ignoring the need to titrate and individualize analgesic doses. The commonly held view that pain is an inevitable and/or insignificant symptom also serves as a barrier to appropriate pain treatment. Some clinicians simply need to be convinced that even though it eventually subsides, pain is a problem.[20]

Fear of addiction, tolerance, side effects. Some clinicians have inaccurate and exaggerated concerns about addiction, tolerance, respiratory depression, and other opioid side effects, which lead them to be extremely cautious about the use of these drugs.[11, 21, 22, 23] This attitude prevails despite the fact there is no evidence that addiction is a significant issue when persons are given opioids for pain control.[24]

Furthermore, many clinicians mistakenly believe that tolerance and physical dependence are synonymous with addiction. They are not. *Tolerance* is a physiologic state resulting from regular use of a drug, in which an increased dosage is needed to produce the same effect, or a reduced effect is observed with a constant dose. Tolerance to the analgesic effects of opioids is not an inevitable consequence of chronic opioid therapy. Experience with treating cancer pain, for instance, has shown that the need for an increase in drug dosage is most likely due to increasing pain caused by progression of the disease. Furthermore, since there is no dose ceiling for most opioids, if tolerance develops, the dose can be increased so long as side effects do not become limiting. *Physical dependence* is a physiologic state of neuro-adaptation characterized by the emergence of a withdrawal syndrome if drug use is stopped or decreased abruptly, or if an antagonist is administered.[25] Physical dependence is an anticipated physiological response even to a short course of opioid therapy. *Addiction,* however, is an abnormal behavioral condition in which a person develops an overwhelming and compulsive involvement in the acquisition and use of a drug for its psychological benefits

and not for medical reasons.[27] Most importantly, when individuals are addicted or psychologically dependent, their quality of life is not improved.

Finally, fear of side effects such as respiratory depression is often cited as a reason to limit opiod use. Although respiratory depression is rare in patients who have been receiving chronic opioid therapy, it is a risk in treating opioid-naive patients with severe pain who require high opioid doses.[63] However, tolerance develops rapidly to the respiratory depressant effects of opioids. Other common side effects of opioids include sedation and nausea, which often subside with continued use.[26] However, since tolerance does not develop to the constipating effects of opioids, this should be anticipated and managed preventively with dietary changes and regular laxative use.

The Organizational Commitment to Pain Management

Consistent with pain management guidelines issued by both the Agency for Healthcare Research and Quality (AHRQ) and the American Pain Society (APS), the Joint Commission stance emphasizes a collaborative and interdisciplinary approach; individualized pain-control plans; assessment and frequent reassessment of patient, resident, or client pain; the use of both pharmacological and nonpharmacological strategies to alleviate pain; and the establishment of a formalized approach to pain management. This systemwide interdisciplinary approach has become known as "institutionalizing pain management." Ideally, it focuses on identifying and breaking down system barriers to effective pain management, while using several methods to incorporate the basic principles of pain management into patterns of daily practice.[27]

The following eight steps, from *Building an Institutional Commitment to Pain Management* by the Wisconsin Cancer Pain Initiative, can serve an organization as it develops and implements its pain management approach.[28]

1. Develop an interdisciplinary workgroup.

2. Analyze current pain management practices in your care setting.

3. Articulate and implement a standard of practice.

4. Establish accountability for pain management.

5. Provide information about pharmacologic and nonpharmacologic intervention to clinicians to facilitate order writing and interpretation and implementation of orders.

6. Promise individuals a quick response to their reports of pain.

7. Provide education for staff.

8. Continually evaluate and work to improve the quality of pain management.

These themes appear throughout this book and in the Joint Commission standards, as they are at the heart of the organizational commitment to better pain management in any health care setting.

The Joint Commission's New Standards

Because the Joint Commission views pain management as an integral component of care, it has expanded the scope of its pain management standards.

Pain management standards apply to organizations involved in the direct provision of care. The new standards, which have been endorsed by the American Pain Society, are published in the 2000 and 2001 editions of the accreditation manuals for organizations involved in the direct provision of care:

- **Ambulatory care;**

- **Behavioral health care;**

- **Home care;**

- **Hospital;**

- **Long term care;**

- **Long term care pharmacy;** and

- **Health care network organizations.**

The new standards acknowledge that while pain coexists with a number of diseases and injuries, it requires explicit attention. Consequently, patients, residents, and clients should be effectively treated for the illness as well as for any associated pain. Overall, the standards require organizations to

- recognize the individual's right to appropriate pain assessment and management;

- identify persons with pain in initial assessments and ongoing (as needed) reassessments; and

- educate patients, residents, and clients and their families about pain management as appropriate.

Standards chapters with new pain management focus. The Joint Commission has inserted a pain management focus in the following six standards chapters:

- **Rights and ethics.** *Recognize the right of individuals to appropriate assessment and management of pain.* This standard represents the organizational commitment to pain management. Health care organizations may make this commitment explicit through their mission statements, patient, resident, client and family bill of rights, or service standards. See Chapter 2 for a more detailed discussion of this standard.

- **Assessment of persons with pain.** *Assess the existence and, if so, the nature and intensity of* *pain in all patients, residents, or clients.* This standard represents the organizational recognition that pain is a common experience and that unrelieved pain has negative consequences. To comply with the standard, the organization incorporates pain assessment into its procedures. It develops procedures for recording assessment results and for ongoing reassessment and follow up. As part of this standard, the organization also determines and assures staff competency in pain assessment and management, and incorporates training on pain assessment and management in the orientation of all new clinical staff. See Chapter 3 for a detailed discussion of this standard.

- **Care of persons with pain.** *Establish policies and procedures that support the appropriate prescribing or ordering of effective pain medications.* This standard asserts that one goal of care is the treating of symptoms that might be associated with a disease, condition, or treatment including pain. In the context of pain management, it focuses on appropriate prescription and administration of patient-controlled analgesia (PCA), spinal-epidural or intravenous medications, and other pain management techniques. A detailed discussion of this standard appears in Chapter 4 of this book.

- **Education of persons with pain.** *Educate patients, residents, and clients and their families about effective pain management.* This standard specifies that the organization is responsible for helping patients, residents, and clients understand the importance of pain management as a part of treatment. In particular, organizations must present individuals with balanced and accurate information on pain medication, as many misconceptions exist for them. A detailed discussion of this standard appears in Chapter 5 of this book.

- **Continuum of care.** *Address the individual's needs for symptom management in the discharge planning process.* The revised standard includes pain as a symptom that should be addressed when considering an individual's needs after discharge. A discussion of this standard appears in Chapter 6 of this book.

- **Improving organization performance.** *Incorporate pain management into the organization's performance measurement and improvement program.* This revised standard specifies that as the organization collects data to monitor its performance, it should consider the appropriateness and effectiveness of its pain management program. Details appear in Chapter 7 of this book.

Chapter 2:

RIGHTS AND ETHICS

This Joint Commission standard addresses the individual's right to involvement in all aspects of his or her care. A health care organization promotes this right by implementing "policies and procedures that are compatible with [its] mission and resources, have diverse input, and guarantee communication across the organization." Furthermore, the organization's leaders and others collaborate to develop, approve, and maintain structures that will promote individual and family involvement in their care. One intent is to encourage individuals to be involved in making care decisions. And in the revised intent statement for this standard, individuals' involvement includes making decisions about managing their pain.

Patient, Resident, and Client Involvement

The Comprehensive Accreditation Manual for Hospitals: The Official Handbook (CAMH) illustrates one way of implementing this standard:

A hospital includes a commitment to pain management in its mission statement, patient and family bill of rights, or service standards (for example, "Patients have the right to expect quick response to reports of pain."). The following is

an example of such a statement posted in all patient care areas at a community hospital:

Patient Rights

As a patient at this hospital, you can expect

- information about pain and pain relief measures;
- a concerned staff committed to pain prevention and management;
- health professionals who respond quickly to reports of pain;
- health professionals who believe your reports of pain; and
- state-of-the-art pain management.

Patient Responsibilities

As a patient at this hospital, we expect that you will

- ask your doctor or nurse what to expect regarding pain and pain management;
- discuss pain relief options with your doctor and nurse;
- work with your doctor and nurse to develop a pain management plan;

- ask for pain relief when pain first begins;

- help your doctor and nurse assess your pain;

- tell your doctor or nurse if your pain is not relieved; and

- tell your doctor or nurse about any worries you have about taking pain medication.

Organizational Support

Health care organizations can promote individual involvement in the ways that best suit their organization. Compliance can be evidenced via the following:

- Interviews with patients, residents, or clients and their families;

- Interviews with organization leaders;

- Interviews with clinical staff;

- Policies and procedures or other processes concerning

  - rights and responsibilities,

  - informed consent,

  - advance directives,

  - research, investigation, or clinical trials,

  - resolution of conflict in care or treatment decisions,

  - withholding resuscitation and forgoing or withdrawing life-sustaining treatment, and

  - pain management; and

- clinical records.

Health care organizations involve individuals in pain management by acknowledging the individual's right to ask for and receive relief from pain. The organization also puts the policies and pro-cedures in place that allow an effective pain management program to develop. Forming an interdisciplinary workgroup to launch the pain management program, assess current pain management policies, and set standards of care is one such procedure.

The interdisciplinary workgroup. As mentioned, many disciplines should cooperate to make pain assessment and management a priority in an organization's day-to-day processes. A pain management workgroup can be formed that includes representatives from all disciplines and settings in which individuals receive care: clinical nurses, nurse educators, physicians, pharmacists, and managers (see Appendix A for Resources for Pain Care Committees and Workgroups 79). Staff nurses involved in direct care should comprise most of the membership, because they know firsthand the problems associated with pain and the barriers to managing it.[27] Among those who could serve as consultants on an as-needed basis are representatives from social services, pastoral care, psychology, and respiratory and occupational/physical therapy. Sometimes a patient, resident, client, or family member is invited to serve on the workgroup.

An organization shows support for such pain management initiatives by having administrative personnel serve on the workgroup or by forming a pain steering committee, which would include chiefs of staff or medical directors and administrators. In addition, organization leaders may show support through their endorsement of an operational budget that finances the time required for staff to attend meetings and classes.[20]

The workgroup can be responsible for the following tasks:

- Defining and implementing standards for pain assessment, documentation, and treatment;

- Making information about analgesics and nonpharmacological strategies readily available;

- Defining accountability for pain management;

- Continuously monitoring and improving the quality of pain management; and

- Providing continuing education opportunities for staff, physicians, patients, residents, and clients. [27, 28]

The organizational needs assessment. One of the workgroup's first assignments should be to perform an institutional needs assessment (see Figure 2.1 for Institutional Assessment of Structures that Support Pain Relief). A needs assessment can help identify an organization's strengths and weaknesses regarding pain management, prioritize the task force's activities, and ensure that important needs are not overlooked. Data collection is central to this needs assessment. An important part of the needs assessment, also, is determining current practices and knowledge of the staff. This can be accomplished through staff testing and focus groups.

Staff testing. Several performance-based assessment tools exist to determine information ranging from general staff knowledge of analgesic pharmacology to beliefs about addiction and various pain-relief methods. Among these tests are the Basic Pain Skills Inventory, the Index of Attitudes About Pain Management, the Pain Control Survey, the Objective Structured Clinical Evaluation, the Knowledge and Attitude Survey Regarding Pain, Nurses' Pain Knowledge and Attitude, and the Cancer Pain Knowledge Inventory. When individuals, particularly clinicians, are confronted with questions they cannot answer, their uncertainty becomes a strong motivator for seeking out further or correct information. [29, 30]

These performance-based assessment tools, which can be tailored to an organization's needs, can be used to perform a variety of activities:

- Identify and prioritize needs;

- Develop a broader institutional needs assessment;

- Develop special one-time educational events and products that address specific knowledge or attitude gaps;

- Match onsite informational products to specific sites of care;

- Develop a whole curriculum for medical, nursing, and pharmacy schools; pain resource nurse programs; preceptorships; and residency rotations in pain management;

- Develop role playing exercises to reveal knowledge and attitude issues prevalent in the organization;

- Adapt pain management guidelines to match the organization's needs;

- Monitor the effectiveness of educational efforts through retesting 12 or 18 months later;

- Revise the test for new groups;

- Define competencies for staff;

- Develop credentialing and privileging policies for licensed independent practitioners; and

- Clarify existing policies and procedures or draft new ones. [31]

Figure 2.1 Institutional Assessment of Structures that Support Pain Relief

	Yes	No
I. Papers (documentation or forms) that support or reinforce standardized pain management:	**Yes**	**No**
1. Do admission forms screen patients for problems with pain?		
2. Are there flow sheets to document the ongoing assessment of pain and the progress toward adequate pain relief? Are these visible to all the members of the health care team?		
3. Are there care plans/protocols/critical paths that identify standard ways to manage different types of pain?		
4. Are there protocols/algorithms that identify strategies to manage analgesic-induced adverse effects (for example, nausea, sedation, constipation)?		
5. Are there medication forms that are readily available and easy to use that support appropriate analgesic administration principles (equianalgesic conversion charts, non-p.r.n. dosing for chronic pain, patient-controlled analgesia [PCA] standards)?		
6. Are there methods to document or signal ongoing, severe, or unrelieved pain (for example, incident reports)?		
II. Educational efforts that provide basic and ongoing education about pain relief strategies:	**Yes**	**No**
1. Are basic pain management principles part of the skills that new staff (nurses/MDs/others) are required to demonstrate competency in before caring for patients?		
2. Are there opportunities for case presentations or rounds on patients with pain problems? Do these cases get as much priority as disease cases?		
3. Are there expert models in pain management that are readily available for staff to adopt into the institution's pain relief ethic?		
4. Is there an interdisciplinary pain consultation service that will evaluate complex pain problems?		
5. Are there resources/classes for patient and family education and how to participate in achieving adequate pain relief?		
III. Institutional policies that support or direct expectations of staff to pursue satisfactory pain relief:	**Yes**	**No**
1. Are there standards/policies for pain assessment, pain intensity thresholds, and triggers for pain consultation or review?		
2. Are there regular measures of patient satisfaction?		
3. Are there policies/procedures that direct the appropriate use of pain technology (for example, PCA pumps, intraspinal infusions, parenteral morphine pumps, infusions)?		
4. Is pain considered an important aspect of care that is monitored through a quality improvement process?		
IV. Innovations that may indicate institutional commitment to recognizing pain as a priority problem:	**Yes**	**No**
1. Are there continuous quality improvement project teams analyzing the systems in place to support adequate pain relief?		
2. Is there research being conducted on strategies to improve pain management?		
3. Is there a pain hot line/consultation service available to outside resources?		
4. Are costs of pain management analyzed?		
5. Is the institution connected to a network or organization concerned about adequate pain relief?		
6. Has the institution ever conducted focus groups of staff or patients to evaluate pain relief?		

Source: Ferrell B, Whedon M, Rollins B. Pain and quality assessment/improvement, *Journal of Nursing Care Quality* 9(3):71, 1995. Reprinted with permission.

Figure 2.2 Examples of Standards for Pain Assessment, Treatment and Documentation

1. Patients will be promised attentive analgesic care by being informed verbally and in writing at the time of their initial interview that effective pain relief is an important part of their treatment, that their report of unrelieved pain is essential, and that staff will respond quickly to their reports of pain.

   → Providing patients with verbal and written information about the institution's promise of attentive analgesic care will be documented in the patient's medical record.

2. Patients will be taught to use a (age-appropriate, condition-appropriate, language-appropriate) pain rating scale to report pain intensity.

   → Teaching patients about the use of the pain rating scale, including the type of scale, will be documented in the patient's medical record.

3. When patients are taught to use the pain rating scale, they will be asked to set a comfort (pain relief) goal. The comfort goal is articulated in terms of function and quality-of-life parameters. In setting the comfort goal, patients will be told that pain rated above the goal (for example, > 3 on scale of 0 to 10) interferes with important activities the patient must be able to perform (such as deep breathing, ambulating, visiting with family) and will trigger an analgesic dose increase, additional analgesic, or other pain relief intervention.

   → The comfort goal and related patient teaching will be documented in the patient's medical record.

4. At the time of initial evaluation and at least once every 8 hours, all patients will be asked about the presence and intensity of pain. The initial pain assessment will include pain quality, location, onset, duration, aggravating and alleviating factors, effects of pain on function and quality of life, and response to past interventions.

   → Initial and subsequent pain assessments will be documented in the patient's medical record.

5. A pain rating greater than the patient's comfort goal will trigger an analgesic dose increase, additional analgesic, or other pain relief intervention.

   → The patient's medical record will show evidence of the use of a pain relief intervention.

6. Pain intensity will be assessed within one hour after a pain relief intervention.

   → The patient's pain rating within one hour after a pain relief intervention will be documented in the patient's medical record.

7. Pain ratings that are persistently above the comfort goal will trigger an interdisciplinary review of the pain management plan and a modification in treatment.

   → The patient's medical record will show evidence of an interdisciplinary review of the pain management plan and a modification in treatment.

Source: Pasero C, et al. *Pain Clinical Manual.* St Louis, MO; Mosby, 1999. Used with permission.

Each group that participates in the assessment testing should receive feedback on its performance. The feedback loop can help the organization and the individuals identify organizational processes that detract from adequate pain management; for example, a lack of standardized pain-assessment tools or skepticism about non-pharmacologic interventions.

Focus groups and other assessment approaches. Conducting focus groups for health care professionals can also determine the level of staff knowledge and elicit continuing education themes. In addition, focus groups provide an outlet for staff, who often need to express their frustrations about the daily management of pain. Those frustrations decrease markedly when there is a constructive outlet for them.[32] Finally, case reviews, drug-use reviews, and medical-record audits can elicit data on medical practices that can be targeted for change, such as inappropriate use of meperidine and the intramuscular (IM) route of administration.[27]

Standards of care. Once the needs assessment is complete, the workgroup should establish standards of care for pain assessment, pain relief, and documentation of both these activities. (See Figure 2.2 for Examples of Standards for Pain Assessment, Treatment, and Documentation.) By implementing standards of care, the task force ensures a common vocabulary for all clinicians who treat persons with pain.[27] Standards of care also help assign accountability and guarantee a uniform system of measurement over time. Guidelines, such as those published by the AHRQ, can be used as a basis for developing such standards of care.[20, 33, 34]

Chapter 3:

ASSESSMENT OF PERSONS WITH PAIN

The goal of an initial pain assessment is to characterize an individual's pain by location, intensity, and etiology. A pain assessment should include a detailed history, physical examination, psychosocial assessment, and diagnostic evaluation. But the single most reliable indicator of the existence and intensity of pain is the individual's self-report. In fact, the individual's report should be the *primary* source of information, since it is more accurate than the observations of others.[35]

The APS guidelines for the treatment of acute and cancer pain suggest that each of the following assessment steps occur:

- The individual's self-report of pain is charted and displayed.

- The intensity of pain and discomfort are assessed and documented at regular intervals (such as prior to medications and then after drugs are administered).

- The degree of pain intensity is measured after allowing sufficient time to pass to ensure peak treatment effect has occurred.[36]

The new Joint Commission standards also highlight the need for a comprehensive assessment of pain in all individuals, if during the initial screening assessment the organization identifies individuals with pain. When the individual is experiencing pain, he or she can be treated within the organization or referred for treatment. The scope of treatment is based on the care setting and services provided. A more comprehensive assessment is performed when warranted by the individual's condition. The results of this more comprehensive assessment, including a measure of pain intensity and quality, are recorded so that regular reassessment and follow up according to criteria developed by the organization can occur.

The Right to Appropriate Assessment

The Joint Commission standard asserts that individuals served "have the right to appropriate assessment and management of pain." The intent acknowledges that although pain can be a common experience, unrelieved pain has adverse physiological and psychological effects. Therefore, staff must respect and support each individual's right to pain management. To fulfill the intent of the standard,

the organization plans, supports, and coordinates activities and resources to ensure that the pain of all individuals is recognized and addressed appropriately. This includes

- initial assessment and regular reassessment of pain;

- education of relevant providers in pain assessment and management;

- education of persons with pain, and families when appropriate, regarding their roles in managing pain as well as the potential limitations and side effects of pain treatments; and

- after considering personal, cultural, spiritual, and ethnic beliefs, communicating to individuals and families that pain management is an important part of care.

An organization can implement this standard in many ways with the goal being that each individual's pain is recognized and treated appropriately. The manual offers several possibilities.

For example, a hospital may determine that every individual should be asked screening questions regarding pain on admission, such as Do you have pain now? Have you had pain in the past several weeks or months?

Or, an organization may consider pain the "fifth" vital sign, meaning that staff would assess and record pain intensity along with temperature, pulse, respiration, and blood pressure, and determine appropriate follow-up care.

In both examples, if the individual says yes, staff explore the following:

- Pain intensity. Use a pain intensity rating scale (example on page 15) appropriate for the individual's age. Pain intensity ratings should be obtained for pain now, at worst, and at best or least. The same pain-rating scales should be used consistently throughout the organization and across disciplines.

- Location. Ask the individual to mark on a diagram or point to the site or sites of pain.

- Quality, patterns of radiation, if any, and character. Elicit and record the individual's own words whenever possible.

- Onset, duration, variation, and patterns.

- Alleviating and aggravating factors.

- Present pain management regimen and effectiveness.

- Pain management history. This includes the individual's medication history, presence of common barriers to reporting pain and using analgesics, past interventions and response, and manner of expressing pain.

- Effects of pain. This includes impact on daily life, function, sleep, appetite, relationships with others, emotions, concentration, and so forth.

- The individual's pain goal. This includes pain intensity and goals related to function, activities, and quality of life.

- Physical examination/observation of the pain site.

Pain Assessment Techniques

The individual's self-report of pain is often measured by using pain scales. A variety of pain scales exist (see Figure 3.1 a, b,c, d—numeric, single descriptive, visual analog, and Wong-Baker FACES). Whichever one is used, it should be reliable, valid, and geared toward the individual, to ensure that it is easy to use and clearly understood. An organization may enlarge and display pain intensity scales in all areas where assessments are conducted.

Numerical pain scales use a 0 to 10 scale to assess the degree of pain. Simple descriptive scales use such word descriptions as "mild," "moderate," and "severe" to describe the patient's

Figure 3.1 Samples of Pain Rating Scales

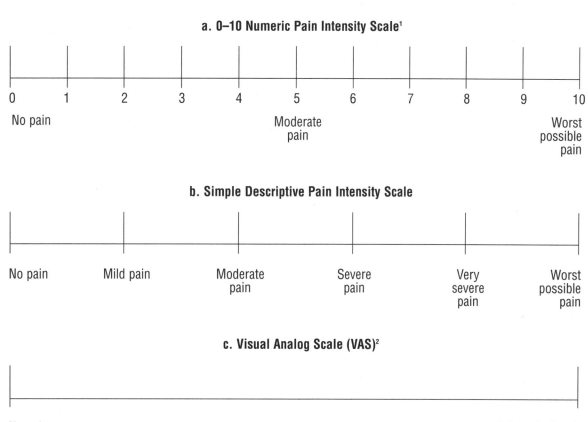

a. 0–10 Numeric Pain Intensity Scale[1]

0   1   2   3   4   5   6   7   8   9   10

No pain   Moderate pain   Worst possible pain

b. Simple Descriptive Pain Intensity Scale

No pain   Mild pain   Moderate pain   Severe pain   Very severe pain   Worst possible pain

c. Visual Analog Scale (VAS)[2]

No pain   Pain as bad as it could possibly be

[1] If used as a graphic rating scale, a 10 cm baseline is recommended.
[2] A 10 cm baseline is recommended for VAS scales.

d. Wong-Baker FACES Pain Rating Scale

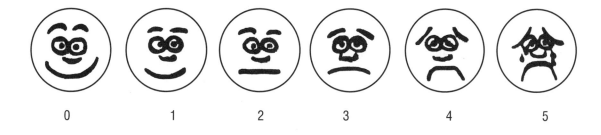

0   1   2   3   4   5

Source, a–c: Acute Pain Management Guideline Panel. *Acute Pain Management: Operatve Medical Procedures and Trauma. Clinical Practice Guideline No. 1* - AHCPR Publication No. 92-0032. Rockville, MD: Agency for Health Care Policy and Research, Feb 1992.

Source, d: Wong DL: *Whaley and Wong's Nursing Care of Infants and Children*, 5th ed. St. Louis, MO, Mosby, 1999. Used with permission.

pain intensity. Visual analogue scales require patients to mark a point on a 10-cm horizontal or vertical line to indicate their pain intensity—zero indicating "no pain" and 10 indicating "the worst possible pain."

In addition to reporting pain intensity, patients should learn that they may have pain in more than one site and they should be encouraged to report as many sites as are relevant, perhaps by pointing to a diagram. All responses should be recorded for future reference.

Often, an organization may need more than one pain intensity scale based on the needs of its various populations. For consistency sake, an organization may select certain pain intensity scales, to use across departments. Before a hospital, clinic, hospice program, or long term care organization decides to adopt one or more pain intensity scales, it should consider developmental stage, chronological age, functional status, cognitive abilities, and emotional status of the populations served.

Adults should be encouraged to use the 0 to 10 numeric scale. If they cannot understand or are unwilling to use it, the smile-frown or the verbal scale can be used. A health care organization serving both children and adults could use two scales, one for each of its populations. A pediatric hospital could include information about pain and pain assessment in its orientation materials for parents, including the parent's role in interpreting behavioral changes of the child that may indicate pain or discomfort.

If clinicians consistently observe discordance between the individuals' verbal self-report of pain and their behaviors and ability to function, staff should conduct further assessment to ascertain the reason for the discordance. It may be due to a variety of causes, such as stoicism, learned coping skills, expectations about how much pain must exist before taking adequate analgesia, previous experience, family dysfunction, or adversarial relationships between the individual, family, and health care team.

When this kind of discordance occurs in a home-care setting, the care provider may want to seek the expertise of an interdisciplinary team, including a chronic disease specialist or representatives from social work or psychology for consultation. A behavioral health organization may want to appoint an interdisciplinary team, including persons knowledgeable in both pain and chemical dependency treatment, a social worker, psychologist, or chronic disease specialist. Because persons with chronic pain can be labeled as "addicted" to their pain medications, a treatment facility for chemical dependency may appoint an interdisciplinary work group or consult recent medical literature and experts on pain and addiction to formulate a policy and process for differentiating between chronic, unrelieved pain, and true chemical dependency.

Assessments Tailored to Distinct Populations

Different populations have different pain, and therefore, different pain assessment and management needs. Five general populations are discussed here the elders, infants and children, persons with cancer or AIDS, persons at the end of life, and adults who have difficulty communicating.

Elders. Many elderly individuals suffer from conditions that are a source of chronic pain, such as arthritis, bone and joint disorders, back problems, gout, and peripheral vascular disease. Many believe that pain is a normal consequence of the aging process. [2, 8, 9, 37] Moreover, many are reluctant to report pain due to ageist attitudes (such as old people complain of pain; they have difficulty using patient-controlled analgesics [PCAs]; they are unreliable pain reporters). [2, 8, 9]

Finally, many fear being perceived as bothersome, a hypochondriac, or an addict. All these attitudes contribute to the likelihood that pain will be undertreated for many elders.[2, 38]

According to clinical practice guidelines for the management of chronic pain in older persons, published by the American Geriatrics Society (AGS), elderly persons who have chronic pain should also be assessed for acute pain, which may indicate that new illnesses are present.[24] These guidelines also address pharmacologic treatments, nonpharmacologic strategies, and recommendations for health systems that care for older persons. Because chronic pain in the elderly is commonly associated with mood disorders, depression, and anxiety, assessments should include an evaluation of psychiatric comorbidity.[39] Figure 3.2, Assessment of Chronic Pain in Older Persons, is a sample of special care guidelines for one particular population.

Infants and children. Pediatric patients are often undertreated for postoperative pain.[40] Part of the reason for undermedication may be that children exhibit and cope with pain differently than adults do. For one, they may be less verbal. For another, they may exhibit a wide range of responses: a child in pain might cry or fuss, make a distressed face, hold or touch the place where it hurts, become very quiet, or sleep excessively.

Pediatric patients may benefit from a preoperative psychosocial assessment to determine their level of distress in anticipation of surgery and their coping history, both of which can affect the amount of postoperative pain they experience.[41] Children who report minimal distress before surgery may have difficulty coping with the pain they experience after surgery. Identifying these children before surgery would enable staff to better prepare and educate the children about surgery and pain.

Staff may also need to use a pain assessment tool designed specifically for children, such as the Wong/Baker Faces Pain Rating Scale, which depicts a series of faces ranging from smiles at the "no hurt" end to tears at the "worst possible hurt" end. But even a faces scale won't help determine an infant's level of pain. Staff must rely on contextual information, diagnosis, and the infant's response to routine comfort measures for determining an infant's pain level.[42] Staff must also learn to assess facial expressions (a grimacing or tense face), body movements (flailing, splinting, kicking, or being still), crying, groaning, and/or changes in vital signs (heart rate and blood pressure). The Barrier and Attia's Observational Instrument and the Modified Infant Pain Scale have been used to accurately assess pain in this age group.[43]

Persons with AIDS; persons with cancer. Although persons with AIDS suffer pain comparable to that of persons with cancer, the former are twice as likely to be undermedicated for pain.[44, 45] One reason is that the focus tends to be on treating potentially reversible problems, such as quelling opportunistic infections, and as a result, pain management may be neglected.[45] In addition, certain drugs that fight the opportunistic infections also cause the neuropathic pain syndromes that HIV-infected persons suffer.

Persons with cancer can have transient pain, long-term pain, or both, related to either the disease or treatment. They also may have unrelated preexisting painful conditions that should be assessed and treated.

Persons at the end of life. There are no data to show that fostering effective pain management for persons at the end of life shortens life. On the other hand, in all instances where the primary intent of therapeutic interventions is to alleviate pain and suffering and not to cause death,

Figure 3.2 Assessment of Chronic Pain in Older Persons

Specific Recommendations

I. On initial presentation of an older person to any health care service, a health care professional should assess the patient for evidence of chronic pain.

II. Persistent or recurrent pain that has a significant impact on function or quality of life should be recognized as a significant problem.

III. A variety of terms synonymous with pain should be used to screen older patients (burning, discomfort, aching, soreness, heaviness, tightness).

IV. For those with cognitive or language impairments, nonverbal pain behavior, recent changes in function, and vocalizations suggest pain as a potential cause (changes in gait, withdrawn or agitated behavior, moaning, groaning, or crying).

V. For those with cognitive or language impairments, reports from a caregiver should be sought.

VI. Conditions that require specific interventions should be identified and treated definitively if possible.

A. Underlying disease should be managed optimally.

B. Patients who need specialized services or skilled procedures should be referred for consultation to a healthcare specialist who has expertise in such services and procedures.

1. Patients identified as having debilitating psychiatric complications should be referred for psychiatric consultation.

2. Patients identified as abusing or as being addicted to any legal or illicit substance should be referred for consultation with an expert who has experience in pain and addiction management.

3. Patients with life-altering intractable pain should be referred to a multidisciplinary pain management center.

VII. All patients with chronic pain should undergo comprehensive pain assessment.

A. Comprehensive pain assessment should include a medical history and physical examination, as well as a review of the results of the pertinent laboratory and other diagnostic tests, with the goals of recording a temporal sequence of events that led to the present pain complaint and establishing a definitive diagnosis, plan for care, and likely prognosis.

B. Initial evaluation of the present pain complaint should include characteristics such as intensity, character, frequency (or pattern, or both), location, duration, and precipitating and relieving factors.

C. Initial evaluation should include a thorough analgesic medication history, including current and previously used prescription medications, over-the-counter medications, and "natural" remedies. The effectiveness and any side effects of current and previously used medications should be recorded.

D. Initial evaluation should include a comprehensive physical examination with particular focus on the neuromuscular system (search for neurologic impairments, weakness, hyperalgesia, hyperpathia, allodynia, numbness, paresthesia) and the musculoskeletal system (palpation for tenderness, inflammation, deformity, trigger points).

Figure 3.2 continued

E. Initial evaluation should include evaluation of physical functions.

    1. Evaluation of physical function should include a focus on pain-associated disabilities, including activities of daily living (Katz ADLs,[60] Lawton IADLs,[61] FIMs,[62] Barthel Index[63]).

    2. Evaluation of physical function should include performance measures of function (range of motion, Up-and-Go Test,[64] Tinetti Gait and Balance Test[65]).

F. Initial evaluation should include evaluation of psychosocial function.

    1. Evaluation of psychosocial function should include assessment of the patient's mood, especially for depression (a geriatric depression scale,[66] CES-D scale[67]).

    2. Evaluation of psychosocial function should include assessment of the patient's social networks, including any dysfunctional relationships.

G. A quantitative assessment of pain should be recorded by the use of a standard pain scale (visual analogue scale, word descriptor scale, numerical scale[58, 68]).

    1. Patients with cognitive or language barriers should be presented with scales that are tailored for their needs and disabilities (scales adapted for speakers of a foreign language, scales in large print, or scales for the visually impaired that do not require visual-spatial skills).

    2. Quantitative estimates of pain based on clinical impressions or surrogate reports should not be used unless the patient is unable to reliably make his or her needs known.

VIII. Patients with chronic pain and their caregivers should be instructed to use a pain log or pain diary with regular entries for pain intensity, medication use, response to treatment, and associated activities.

IX. Patients with chronic pain should be reassessed regularly for improvement, deterioration, or complications attributable to treatment. The frequency of follow-up should be a function of the severity of the pain syndrome and the potential for adverse effects of treatment.

A. Reassessment should include evaluation of significant issues identified in the initial evaluation.

B. The same quantitative assessment scales should be used for follow-up assessments.

C. Reassessment should include an evaluation of analgesic medication use, side effects, and adherence problems.

D. Reassessment should include an evaluation of the positive and negative effects of a nonpharmacologic treatments.

Adapted from: The management of chronic pain in older persons. *Journal of the American Geriatrics Society* 46(7):635–51, May 1998.

aggressive pain management is ethical and appropriate. When pain and suffering are resistant to treatment, sedation may be therapeutic and medically appropriate to provide relief if it is consistent with the wishes of the individual.[46]

Individuals with difficulty communicating. Adults who have difficulty communicating their pain require special considerations. In this group are persons with cognitive or sensory impairments and functional deficits as well as those who are psychotic, severely emotionally disturbed, comatose, or ventilator-dependent; who inadvertently deny pain; who cannot verbally communicate pain; or who do not speak English.

As with infants and children, cognitively impaired persons may signal pain or discomfort via behavioral factors, and staff will need to become attuned to these. A long term care organization caring for persons with Alzheimer's disease may develop a pain scale appropriate to residents with dementia based on the longstanding knowledge of this population as well as common pain syndromes in elderly persons.

Assessment and Reassessment

Pain should be assessed and reassessed at regular intervals to ensure that the individual's pain is being relieved. For acute-pain persons who have just had surgery, the frequency of assessment can be based on the type of surgery performed and the severity of pain. For example, pain should be assessed every two hours during the first postoperative day following major surgery. The frequency of reassessments should be increased if the pain is poorly controlled or the intervention is being changed.

For individuals with chronic pain, such as from cancer or arthritis, a clinician should evaluate the pain every time he or she assesses the individual. In subsequent assessments the clinician should evaluate the effectiveness of the management plan and, if pain has not been relieved, determine whether the pain is related to the progression of disease, to a new cause, or to the treatment. For example, pain could be assessed 15 to 30 minutes after parenteral drug therapy has been administered or one hour after oral medication has been given. In any case, the assessment of the individual's pain and of the efficacy of the treatment plan should be ongoing, and the details of the assessment should be documented.

Documentation of Pain Management

Like assessment, documentation of pain management is often inadequate.[47, 48] The two activities have an important connection because if pain is not perceived to be important enough to document, it probably is not being accurately assessed.[49] However, inadequate documentation can seriously interfere with care and have legal implications.

Documentation techniques. Documentation should cover the type of pain (cancer, arthritic, postoperative); the individual's rating of pain on a pain intensity scale; the individual's level of consciousness, respiratory rate, and activity; the presence of side effects or alternate therapy; the medication regimen; and the extent of patient, resident, or client and family education on pain management.[50] The degree of pain relief should be documented 30 minutes after parenteral analgesic and one hour after oral analgesic administration.

One way to improve documentation is to put a mechanism in place that will ensure that pain is consistently assessed. For example, as mentioned earlier, pain can be adopted as the "fifth vital sign" and, as such, recorded along with the individual's temperature, pulse, respiration, and blood pressure. The concept of pain as the fifth vital sign, originally promoted by the APS to elevate awareness of pain treatment among health care professionals, is gaining wide acceptance in the medical community. The APS maintains that if pain were assessed and recorded with the same zeal as other vital signs, it would have a much better chance of being treated properly.

Some organizations develop protocols/pathways, algorithms, or policies and procedures to ensure that pain management assessment and documentation become as routine as measuring vital signs. [33, 52] Beginning in 1999, the Veterans Health Administration adopted a systemwide protocol that pain be routinely assessed as the fifth vital sign in every individual. In addition, some organizations are beginning to record the presence or absence of pain routinely, and if pain is present, to document its severity.[17] When organizations use assessment scales designed to describe and measure pain, they promote consistent documentation of both pharmacological and nonpharmacological methods for pain relief.[36] Moreover, if clinicians document the pain experience when it occurs rather than at the end of a shift, they may be more likely to comply with documentation protocols.[47]

A host of national organizations have published clinical practice guidelines, standards of care, and consensus statements that could serve as a basis for developing internal documents. Foremost are the AHRQ guidelines, which address the management of acute and postoperative pain in adults and children, cancer pain, and acute back pain. Other organizations, such as the APS and the AAPM have published a consensus statement on the use of opioids for chronic pain; the AGS has published guidelines for the management of chronic pain in older persons; and the WHO published principles for pain relief for children with cancer.

One documentation option is a comprehensive pain flowsheet to assess, monitor, document, and evaluate clients at risk for and/or experiencing pain. This sheet, which can be incorporated into the individual's chart, increases consistency in documentation of pain management activities.[50] Use of the flowsheet can be initiated on admission if the individual's pain is uncontrolled or if the individual is being admitted for a primary diagnosis of pain. If the individual's pain increases, the flowsheet will reflect this and follow the individual's progress throughout the length of service.

Another option is to include a drug chart in the clinical record as a reminder to assess and document pain management.[49] The chart can include a place for a pain rating scale and a place for notes. In fact, research supports the finding that when pain assessment information is included in clinical charts, those individuals' analgesics are more likely to be increased, and those individuals are more likely to report a decrease in number of days with pain.[51]

Overcoming resistance to documentation initiatives. An organization may add a pain management section to the medical chart, to prompt clinicians to record daily outcomes, pharmacological therapies, and nonpharmacological interventions. Another organization may develop a pain-related flowchart that, once completed, will enable the organization to detect patterns in assessment, intervention, and response to intervention over time,[20] or to track individual's pain status.[34] Other new or revised procedures may require the clinician to educate the patient or initiate PCA to prevent the occurrence of breakthrough pain.[52]

Although such strategies have proven effective, they can also backfire, if they create extra steps considered to be burdensome [27] or administrative intrusions on individual practice. Thus, it may be better to introduce changes gradually for example, starting out with a simple alteration to order forms to encourage the use of a preferred analgesic.

The key to using any of these tools is to evaluate them after a specified period of time to determine if clinicians find them helpful or rigid. [19] For example, one organization tried using a vital-sign sheet to screen for the presence and intensity of pain. However, the staff members did not use it initially because they did not understand its purpose. [32] They thought it was intended to replace a full assessment and, as such, was insufficient and duplicative. Once the purpose was clarified, compliance increased.

Staff Education

As noted, health care providers may often perform incomplete pain assessments. They may not ask about the patient's pain history, pattern of pain, or pain intensity. [19] Thus, efforts to change professional practices must focus on getting caregivers to both assess pain and document pain intensity ratings in the clinical record. Staff education about assessment is a critical component of pain management and an important way an organization shows its commitment to pain management.

Exploring educational methods and content. Health care organizations have several options for staff education. During orientation sessions, they can determine the competency of all new clinical staff with regard to pain assessment and treatment. Or the organization can hold twice-annual staff-awareness events regarding pain management topics. Information could also be provided at grand rounds, monthly or quarterly staff meetings, mandatory in-service training for new employees, formal staff in-services, and monthly discussion groups.

A useful approach is to have staff take a brief pretest on key points to be covered during a learning session. Completing a posttest after the session helps participants see how much they've learned and demonstrates which areas need further attention. If these tests are to be useful, participants should receive quick feedback on their performance. Comparing results of pre- and posttesting can reveal the efficacy of educational programs. [19] Pre- and posttest results can also serve as a guide to developing future educational topics, such as the following:

- Pharmacologic treatments, including types of medications, dosing recommendations, routes of administration, and conversion instructions;

- Nonpharmacologic interventions, including physical therapies and cognitive behavioral techniques;

- Effective assessment tools;

- Myths regarding analgesic addiction, tolerance, and side effects;

- The truth about regulatory oversight;

- Special needs of specific populations;

- The importance of the self-report;

- Individual barriers to reporting pain and taking medications;

- The use of opioids for nonmalignant, chronic pain; and

- The role of the pain resource nurse.

The subject of individual barriers to reporting pain and using analgesics is a particularly important one. For example, staff could learn how to encourage the reporting of pain when an individual demonstrates reluctance to discuss it, denies pain when it is likely to be present (for example, following surgery, a trauma, burns, or a cardiac emergency), or does not follow through with recommended treatments.

Pain-related topics can be covered in staff newsletters and displayed on posters and flyers. Handouts for staff could include copies of pertinent guidelines, algorithms, consensus statements, and even a resource list for gathering more information. (See Appendix A for Resource Lists.) Experiential exercises, such as videotaped role play, can be used to effectively update staff pain management skills.[53]

Although lectures, conferences, presentations, and the like are valuable forms of education, learning that occurs on the units is most likely to bring changes in clinical practice.[18, 19, 54] This can occur during weekly pain rounds or during daily guidance from nurses specially trained in pain management.

The Joint Commission standards on assessment suggest that as part of its educational effort, an organization post a statement on pain management for staff in all care areas—patient or resident rooms, clinic rooms, and waiting rooms. The statement may read as follows:

As all individuals have a right to pain relief, staff should

- inform individuals at the time of their initial evaluation that relief of pain is an important part of their care and respond quickly to reports of pain;

- ask individuals on initial evaluation and as part of regular assessments about the presence, quality, and intensity of pain and use the individual's self-report as the primary indicator of pain;

- work together with the individual and other health care providers to establish a goal for pain relief and develop and implement a plan to achieve that goal; and

- review and modify the plan of care for patients who have unrelieved pain.

Reminder tools, too, can help staff practice effective pain management. For example, concise guidelines for analgesic use can be posted on coat-pocket cards given to clinicians and staff or secured to desks on which physicians write orders; guidelines that indicate drug timing and doses can be included in drug order sheets, and computer "help screens" with analgesic equivalency tables can be added to the computerized drug ordering system [19] or pharmacy computer. To remind staff to ask about pain, stickers depicting "faces in pain" can be placed on clinical charts; coat-pocket cards can list 10 key points critical to managing individual pain; and a summary sheet of individuals' pain scales or a checklist indicating appropriate assessment steps can be placed in the charts.[55] In addition, other health care professionals, such as physical therapists, social workers, and dietitians can be trained to help identify persons in pain and to either alert or remind the nurse or physician to assess individuals for pain.

Preceptorships. Another educational technique is the *preceptorship* program in pain management. These programs, designed for clinicians, typically last a few days and include formal lectures, patient rounds and interaction, observation of procedures, contact with departments and disciplines involved in the delivery of pain management services, group discussions, and problem solving. (See Appendix B for information on Preceptorships and Pain Resource Nurse Programs.) [27] Sometimes preceptorship faculty work as mentors with the participants to identify specific goals of practice change (starting a pain assessment program), to identify the barriers to change (lack of administrative support), and help to develop a strategy for beginning the change process at their organizations (forming a pain assessment task force using a QI model).[56]

One example of a preceptorship is the Network Project, established in 1992 by the Pain, Psychiatry, and Rehabilitation Medicine Services of the Departments of Neurology and Psychiatry at Memorial Sloan-Kettering Cancer Center through a grant from the National Cancer Institute. In 1998, the Network Project expanded through collaboration with the newly developed Department of Pain Medicine and Palliative Care at Beth Israel Medical Center in New York City. Today, nearly 400 postgraduate clinicians have participated in the Network Project's two-week observership program. When they return to their own health care organization, participants have an increased knowledge of pain management and psychosocial issues related to cancer and cancer pain, and many bring back new attitudes toward cancer pain issues.[18]

Focusing the educational program. Whether the topic is pharmacologics or documentation, staff education should include all staff members. All key staff members, which includes physicians, nurses, pharmacists, and administration, need to receive the same education to ensure that consistent information is being provided. For example, educational efforts may prompt physicians and nurses to use more opioids and other analgesics as well as investigate alternative routes of administration. But a pharmacist who is not included in the training and who lacks knowledge of pain management may misunderstand this increased use of opioids.[54] On the other hand, a pharmacist can serve as a key figure in educating other staff and even patients, particularly with regard to the pharmacological effects of pain medications and other adjuvant drugs. Administrators can help when educational efforts involve a change in policy, and thus require administrative approval. For example, an organi-

zation may choose to make pain scales consistent across all departments and then provide education for all staff and patients. An administrator can facilitate such a change.

Other staff, such as dietitians, physical therapists, and occupational therapists, who provide direct care to patients should also be involved in pain management education to ensure that their interventions are optimally effective. For example, a dietitian working with an individual who is unable to eat should know which pain medications can impact appetite. Rehabilitation staff should be aware of when the individual is at his or her physical best to participate in therapeutic activities.

A facility may also establish a resident care team to oversee pain assessment and management, and to that end, the team may develop criteria to identify persons with pain or at risk for pain. As a result, every resident is asked about pain on admission. A consultant pharmacist at a long term care pharmacy can assist a long term care facility client to develop pain assessment criteria, participate in the facility's pain management activities, identify residents in need of pain management, and provide information on appropriate drug therapy for pain as part of the drug regimen review.

Benefiting from experts and leaders in pain management. An *opinion leader* in a health care organization is someone who peers trust to evaluate new clinical information, assess new practices, and then determine their value within the context of the local setting. Opinion leaders are not necessarily innovators or authority figures, but once they adopt an innovation, other staff members tend to accept it. An opinion leader who is willing to champion good pain relief is of value, then, to an organization trying to implement a new program. The opinion leader's role is to convince health care providers that their current practices are outdated, inappropriate, unsupported by research evidence, or no longer accepted by colleagues.

The *expert leader,* in contrast, may engage in academic detailing, a type of social-influence strategy for implementing protocols and policies with individuals or in small groups. Academic detailing strategies include conducting interviews to determine baseline knowledge, stimulating active participation during educational sessions, using concise graphic educational materials, and highlighting or replicating essential messages.[57] The practice is modeled after drug detailing, in which representatives of pharmaceutical companies visit physicians to talk about medications in their specialty areas.

If no pain management experts are on staff, however, a clinical nurse specialist in oncology, surgery, or critical care or a nurse anesthetist may take on the role of resident expert. In many health care organizations, a clinical pharmacist has taken on the role of pain management expert. Another option is to bring in an expert from outside the organization to train a small group to serve as resource personnel for other staff nurses. [54]

The concept of the pain resource nurse is gaining popularity at organizations across the country. Responsibilities of pain resource nurses include serving as role models, providing pain management education and consultations, and acting as agents for change.[27] Similar to the pain-resource-nurse program is the nurse-based PCA program, which expands the role of the bedside nurse into the patient's primary pain manager.[27] These specially trained nurses staff the hospital 24 hours a day, serving as resources to bedside nurses in managing patients receiving PCAs. This nurse is also responsible for educating patients before pain therapy is initiated, and ensuring smooth initiation of pain therapy for postoperative patients in the postanesthesia care unit and for nonsurgical patients on the clinical units. Some hospitals have a pain team that serves as a resource to others as well as treats patients or consults under referral. Similar approaches have been implemented in long term care and home care agencies.

Educational interventions have spawned many benefits in health care organizations:

- Significant improvement in staff knowledge related to pain management;

- Increased overall individual satisfaction;[51, 52, 58]

- Increased consistency in individuals' ability to rate their own pain intensity and/or identify their perceived "acceptable" level of pain;

- More consistent patterns of pain management practice by nursing staff;[52, 58]

- Decreased duration of services due to unrelieved pain;[59] and

- Improved compliance with standards of care,[33] including assessment and documentation.

Educational efforts have also significantly altered prescription practices. [51, 60] A key component of these efforts is that staff is exposed to correct information over a period of time; and the longer the time, the better their knowledge level becomes. [61]

Chapter 4:

CARE OF PERSONS WITH PAIN

Joint Commission standards require that organizations provide "individualized care in settings responsive to specific needs. Individuals deserve care that respects their choices, supports their participation in the care provided, and recognizes their right to achieve their personal health goals." The goals of care are met when certain processes are performed well. One process now included in the standard is the treating of symptoms that might be associated with a disease, condition, or treatment, including pain.

Care activities, the standard asserts, "may be carried out by medical, nursing, pharmacy, dietary, rehabilitation, and other types of providers. Each provider's role and responsibility are determined by his or her professional skills, competence, and credentials; the care or rehabilitation being provided; (organization) policies; and relevant licensure, certification, regulation, privileges, scope of practice, or job description."

The standards on care also address pain in the context of rehabilitation services, defined as services designed to help individuals "achieve an optimal level of functioning, independence, and quality of life." Here, the standards recognize that pain may keep individuals from reaching optimal functioning and, thus, should be identified during the assessment process and incorporated into the care planning process.

The *Comprehensive Accreditation Manual for Ambulatory Care* gives this example of implementation:

> In a day surgery setting, discharge criteria are set, including pain, that determines if an individual is ready for discharge to home. The day surgery center also contacts the individual the following day. One of the assessment parameters asked of the individual, depending on the surgical procedure, includes changes in pain intensity, relief from prescribed medications, and ability to rest. Based on the results of the assessment, follow up is initiated per the day surgery protocols.

Although much of the standard focuses on the safe and appropriate prescription and monitoring of controlled medications, a growing body of literature supports the effectiveness of several non-phamacological treatments for pain (see Figure 4.1, Scientific Evidence for Interventions to Manage Pain in Adults). The following two sections give brief overviews of these topics.

Figure 4.1 Scientific Evidence for Interventions to Management Pain in Adults

Pharmacologic Interventions

Interventions[1]		Type of Evidence	Comments
NSAIDs	Oral (alone)	Ib.IV	Effective for mild to moderate pain. Begin preoperatively. Relatively contraindicated in patients with renal disease and risks of or actual coagulopathy. May mask fever.
	Oral (adjunct to opioid	Ia.IV	Potentiating effect resulting in opioid) sparing. Begin preop. Cautions as above.
	Parenteral (ketorolac)	Ib.IV	Effective for moderate to severe pain. Expensive. Useful where opioids contraindicated, especially to avoid respiratory depression and sedation. Advance to opioid.
Opioids	Oral	IV	As effective as parenteral in appropriate doses. Use as soon as oral medication tolerated. Route of choice.
	Intramuscular	Ib.IV	Has been the standard parenteral route, but injections painful and absorption unreliable. Hence, avoid this route when possible.
	Subcutaneous	Ib.IV	Preferable to intramuscular for low-volume continuous infusion. Injections painful and absorption unreliable. Avoid this route for long-term repetitive dosing.
	Intravenous	Ib.IV	Parenteral route of choice after major surgery. Suitable for titrated bolus or continuous administration (including PCA), but requires monitoring. Significant risk of respiratory depression with inappropriate dosing.
	PCA (Systemic)	Ia.IV	Intravenous or subcutaneous routes recommended. Good, steady level of analgesia. Popular with patients but requires special infusion pumps and staff education. See cautions about opioids above.
	Epidural and intrathecal	Ia.IV	When suitable, provides good analgesia. Significant risk of respiratory depression, sometimes delayed in onset. Requires careful monitoring. Use of infusion pumps requires additional equipment and staff education.
Local Anesthetics	Epidural and intrathecal	Ia.IV	Limited indications. Expensive if infusion pumps employed. Effective regional analgesia. Opioid sparing. Addition of opioid to local anesthetic may improve analgesia. Risks of hypotension, weakness, numbness. Use of infusion pump requires additional equipment and staff.
	Peripheral nerve block	Ia.IV	Limited indications and duration of action. Effective regional analgesia. Opioid sparing.

Figure 4.1 continued

Nonpharmacologic Interventions

Intervention[1]		Type of Evidence	Comments
Simple Relaxation (begin preoperatively)	Jaw relaxation Progressive muscle relaxation Simple imagery	Ia. IIa. IIb. IV	Effective in reducing mild to moderate pain and as an adjunct to analgesic drugs for severe pain. Use when patients express interest in relaxation. Requires 3-5 minutes of staff time for instructions.
	Music	Ib, IIa, IV	Both patient-preferred and "easy listening" music are effective in reducing mild to moderate pain.
Complex Relaxation (begin preoperatively)	Biofeedback	Ib, IIa, IV	Effective in reducing mild to moderate pain and operative site muscle tension. Requires skilled personnel and special equipment.
	Imagery	Ib, IIa, III, IV	Effective for reduction of mild to moderate pain. Requires skilled personnel.
Education/ Instruction (begin preoperatively)		Ia, IIa, IIb, IV	Effective for reduction of pain. Should include sensory and procedural information and instruction aimed at reducing activity related pain. Requires 5-15 minutes of staff time.
TENS		Ia, IIa, III, IV	Effective in reducing pain and improving physical function. Requires skilled personnel and special equipment. May be useful as an adjunct to drug therapy.

[1] Insufficient scientific evidence is available to provide specific recommendations regarding the use of hypnosis, acupuncture, and other physical modalities for relief of postoperative pain.

Type of Evidence — Key

Ia	Evidence obtained from meta-analysis of randomized controlled trials.
Ib	Evidence obtained from at least one randomized controlled trial.
IIa	Evidence obtained from at least one well-designed controlled study without randomization.
IIb	Evidence obtained from at least one other type of well-designed quasi-experimental study.
III	Evidence obtained from well-designed nonexperimental descriptive studies, such as comparative studies, correlational studies, and case studies.
IV	Evidence obtained from expert committee reports or opinions and/or clinical experiences of respected authorities.

Source: Acute Pain Management Guideline Panel. *Acute Pain Management: Operative or Medical Procedures and Trauma. Clinical Practice Guideline No. 1.* AHCPR Pub. No. 92-0032. Rockville, MD: Agency for Health Care Policy and Research, Public Health Service, U.S. Department of Health and Human Services. More complete references are available in the *Guideline Report* for this guideline (AHCPR Publication No. 92-0022). Note: Selected references are included in the guideline.

Pharmacological Treatment

Staff should be educated about analgesic pharmacology and pain therapy. The three major classes of drugs that are used alone or, more commonly, in combination to manage pain are non-opioids, opioid analgesics, and adjuvant analgesic agents (see Appendix B for "The Use of Opioids for the Treatment of Chronic Pain" a consensus statement from the AAPM and the APA). Pharmacologic management of pain is a complex topic, however, and beyond the scope of this book. The American Pain Society, the Agency of HealthCare Research and Quality, the American Geriatric Society, and the American Society of Anesthesiologists have developed clinical practice guidelines for pain management, and all are useful sources on this topic.[24, 62, 63, 64, 65, 66] The World Health Organization (WHO) has developed a three-step hierarchy for analgesic pain management, called the Analgesic Ladder. (See Figure 4.2, the WHO Three-Step Analgesic Ladder.)

The Joint Commission standard is that an organization's "policies and procedures support safe medication prescription or ordering." The manuals give several examples of organizational compliance with this standard, including having policies and procedures in place that address prescribing or ordering, procuring, storing, controlling, preparing, and dispensing of medications. In scoring an organization's performance on this standard, surveyors will be concerned with whether procedures address, among other issues, "as needed" (PRN) and scheduled prescriptions, or orders and times of dose administration. Surveyors will also note whether the organization has procedures for "patient-controlled analgesia (PCA), spinal/epidural or intravenous administration of medications, and other pain management techniques in the care of individuals with pain."

The manual gives this example of implementation of the standard on safe medication procedures:

Before initiating PCA for surgical patients, an interdisciplinary team of physicians, pharmacists, and nurses performs the following activities:

- Evaluates drug delivery devices;

- Reviews the medical literature on PCA;

- Drafts policies, procedures, and standing orders;

- Obtains approval from the pharmacy and therapeutics committee and medical staff;

- Orients all staff; and

- Conducts a pilot test on the general surgery care unit.

In a long term care facility, consulting pharmacists should monitor resident records and physician orders to assure, for example, that only one sustained-release opioid is prescribed at a time and that meperidine use is avoided. If either of these situations occurs, the pharmacist would either contact the physician directly or coordinate with nursing staff, and then take the opportunity to educate physicians and nurses about appropriate and safe medication use.

The Joint Commission standards in the Care chapters also instruct that the individual "is monitored during the postprocedural period." Monitoring should focus on, among other things, drugs administered and "pain intensity and quality (for example, pain character, frequency, location, duration) and responses to treatments."

In many organizations, standing orders may cover pain assessment, medication type, dosing, side-effect prevention, and discontinuation of therapy. But algorithms may be designed to guide staff through such activities as continuous infusion for morphine or hydromorphone, conversion from continuous infusion to oral administration, management of painful bone

Figure 4.2 The WHO Three-Step Analgesic Ladder

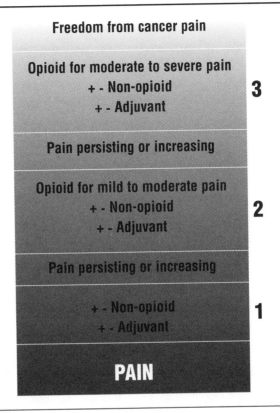

Freedom from cancer pain

Opioid for moderate to severe pain
+ - Non-opioid
+ - Adjuvant
3

Pain persisting or increasing

Opioid for mild to moderate pain
+ - Non-opioid
+ - Adjuvant
2

Pain persisting or increasing

+ - Non-opioid
+ - Adjuvant
1

PAIN

Adapted from: Reproduced by permission of WHO, from *Cancer Pain Relief,* 2nd ed. Geneva: World Health Organization 1996.

metastases, and management of neuropathic pain.[20]

Nonpharmacologic Therapy

Nonpharmacological therapies can also play an important role in pain management. Such nonpharmacologic interventions, used in combination with appropriate drug regimens, often improve overall pain management by enhancing the therapeutic effects of medications and permitting lower dosages to be used.[24, 67, 68] The use of these therapies also reduces the potential for medication side effects.[8] However, although nonpharmacologic interventions may reduce the need for drugs, they should not be used as substitutes for them.[68]

Typically nonpharmacologic interventions are divided into two categories: physical interventions and cognitive behavioral techniques. Physical interventions include cutaneous stimulation, such as the application of heat, cold, or transcutaneous electrical nerve stimulation (TENS); exercise; physical and/or occupational therapy; immobilization; chiropractic; massage; and acupuncture. The National Institutes of Health now recognizes the benefit of acupuncture as an adjunct treatment for painful conditions such as postoperative pain, myofascial pain, low back pain, stroke rehabilitation, headache, menstrual cramps, fibromyalgia, osteoarthritis, and tennis elbow.[67]

Cognitive behavioral strategies are aimed at altering belief structures, attitudes, and thoughts to modify the patient's experience of pain and suffering.[24] These strategies include various forms of distraction, relaxation, guided imagery, biofeedback, and hypnosis. Components include education, coping-skills training, and relapse prevention. If individuals can think differently about their pain, the theory goes, they may gain a sense of control over it [35] and even diminish the pain.[24]

Chapter 5:

EDUCATION OF PERSONS WITH PAIN

Persons with pain as well as staff who care for these people need to be educated about effective pain management. The goal of educating individuals and their families is to involve them in the pain management plan. The Joint Commission standard is that individuals "are taught that pain management is a part of treatment." The intent of this standard is that "staff offer education to individuals and families to give them the specific knowledge and skills they need to meet the patient's ongoing health care needs. Clearly, such instruction needs to be presented in ways that are understandable to those receiving it." Designing appropriate instruction begins with understanding commonly held attitudes about pain treatment.

In general, research supports the idea that Americans would rather bear pain than take actions to relieve it, fearing addiction, dependence on drugs, and tolerance to medications.[69] These beliefs and attitudes affect individuals' willingness to report pain and to use adequate amounts of analgesics to control it.[32, 70] In addition, individuals may underreport pain because they do not want to appear ill informed or unable to understand information pertaining to medication.[71] Finally, many individuals are reluctant to take pain medications, such as opioids,

because they fear they will be unable to function normally.[68] The problem with underreporting of pain is that the pain goes untreated.

The Joint Commission intent statement points out that openness and flexibility are important elements in education openness to individuals' attitudes, needs, abilities, and readiness for education. Thus, staff members must take into account such variables as the patient's and family's

- beliefs and values;

- literacy, educational level, and language;

- emotional barriers and motivations;

- physical and cognitive limitations; and

- the financial implications of care choices.

Educational Content: What Should Be Taught

Patients, residents, and clients can benefit from a structured educational program. Such programs can contribute to decreases in pain intensity, in perceptions of pain severity, in fears of addiction, and in anxiety. They also contribute to increased use of appropriate pain medications [72, 73] and increased pain control. Research supports the idea that individuals who expect pain relief and

Figure 5.1 Facts About Cancer Pain Treatment

If you are being treated for cancer pain, you may have concerns about your treatment. Here are some common concerns and facts about them.

Concern: I can only take medication or other treatments when I have pain.

Fact: You should not wait until the pain becomes severe to take your medication. Pain is easier to control when it is mild than when it is severe. You should take your pain medicine regularly and as your doctor or nurse tells you. This may mean taking it on a regular schedule and around the clock. You can also use the other treatments, such as relaxation and breathing exercises, hot and cold packs, as often as you want.

Concern: I will become "hooked" on or "addicted" to pain medicine.

Fact: Studies show that getting "hooked" or "addicted" to pain medicine is very rare. Remember, it is important to take pain medicine regularly to keep pain under control.

Concern: If I take too much medicine, it will stop working.

Fact: The medicine will not stop working. But sometimes the body will get used to the medicine. This is called tolerance. Tolerance is not usually a problem with cancer pain treatment because the amount of medicine can be changed or other medicines can be added. Cancer pain can be relieved, so don't deny yourself pain relief now.

Concern: If I complain too much, I am not being a good patient.

Fact: Controlling your pain is an important part of your care. Tell your doctor or nurse if you have pain, if your pain is getting worse, or if you are taking pain medicine and it is not working. They can help you get relief from the pain.

You may have concerns about treatment that were not discussed here. Talk to your doctor or nurse about your concerns.

Source: Rischer JB, Childress SB. Cancer pain management; Pilot implementation of the AHCPR guideline in Utah. *Joint Commission Journal on Quality Improvement* 22(10):690, Oct 1996. Originally developed by Health Insight, Salt Lake City, UT. Adapted from Jacox P, et al. *Management of Cancer Pain. Clinical Practice Guideline No. 9.* AHCPR Publication No. 94-0592. Rockville, MD: Agency of Health Care Policy and Research, Mar 1994.

know how to request it are more likely to have better pain control. Such benefits have been seen in clinics that routinely assess and treat pain.[18]

Pain education can begin at the initial evaluation, when an organization informs all individuals and their families that effective pain relief is an important part of treatment. Staff may do this both verbally and in an electronic or printed format. A long term care facility may discuss commonly held myths about pain and aging in educational materials about pain management that it provides to all residents. A long term care pharmacy can provide both in-service education and written materials related to pain assessment and management for staff at its client facilities. A behavioral health organization may prepare an educational packet that includes information about pain and its debilitating effects, ways individuals can communicate pain experience to health care providers, and treatment options. This packet could also include definitions of physical dependence, tolerance, and addiction.

Given that the most reliable indicator of pain is the individual's self-report, education efforts should highlight information about the nature of pain and how to use pain assessment instruments, including pain intensity scales (see chapter 3). Individuals should also be taught to report changes in the nature or degree of pain and the onset of new pain so that appropriate reassessment and change in treatment can be initiated. In addition, individuals should be informed about the harmful effects of unrelieved pain, to encourage them to communicate pain. All individuals and families should know who they can contact when they are in need of pain relief.[27]

Individuals can also be educated about pharmacological and nonpharmacological treatments, including how to manage them. Education in the safe and effective use of medication should include instruction in at least the name and description of the medication; the dosage, route of administration, and duration of drug therapy; the risk of pain and the importance of effective pain management; adverse effects or drug interactions; and prescription or refill information. Support materials should address the issues of addiction and tolerance, and the potential for readdiction in recovering drug users, to correct individuals' misconceptions. Figure 5.1, Facts about Cancer Pain Treatment, is one example of a sensitive education effort.

As part of its pain management improvement initiative, a home care agency may provide information to all clients and their families about common reasons why individuals hesitate to report pain and use analgesics. Then, based on the reason for admission and the scope of services provided, additional information can be given that addresses a patient's specific needs and the organization's policies and processes regarding handling uncontrolled pain.

Similarly, hospital staff can tailor information to a patient's specific pain management needs based on the reason for admission—for example, labor or postoperative pain. In addition, staff may provide follow-up information on managing pain at home, including when to contact the health care provider for further assistance upon discharge or transfer to another health care facility. A hospital may also conduct telephone follow-up interviews concerning, for example, outpatient surgery, short stay obstetrics, or discharge planning, in which staff asks about the patient's pain status.

Recognizing the impact uncontrolled pain has on a patient's functioning, a rehabilitation hospital may decide to distribute information about pain management to all individuals at discharge. This information may include general information about pain; use of medications; use of nonpharmacological interventions, including heat, cold, exercise, and physical therapy; and recommendations on when to call a health care professional for additional assistance.

A comprehensive resident and family education program for a long term care facility, home care agency, or behavioral health organization should include the following:

A General Overview

- Informing the resident that pain can be relieved;

- Identifying the causes of pain;

- Explaining the use of a pain rating scale to assess and communicate pain;

- Explaining the use of diaries to record pain occurrences, intensity, times of medication administration, and relief;

- Encouraging the individual to talk to doctors and nurses about pain and pain management; and

- Introducing a preventive approach to pain control.

Nonpharmacological Management Material

- Discussing deep breathing, relaxation, imagery, distraction, calming self-statements, heat/cold, massage, and exercise.

Health Care System Issues

- Explaining effective self-advocacy skills and behaviors for obtaining pain relief.

Educational Methods: How to Teach Pain Management

If possible, individuals should receive some education before admission. At admission, individuals tend to feel anxious and may have difficulty retaining information. Thus, for example, an ambulatory facility may opt to mail printed educational materials about pain to all individuals before the day of surgery. However, medical literature indicates that to have the desired effect, individual and family information should be presented more than once and in more than one way, so this initial mailing may not be sufficient.

Educational sessions, which can address patients, caregivers, or both, can be conducted one-on-one or in small groups. Information presented in such sessions must be understandable to the individual receiving it, considering the nature of the illness and the constraints it imposes.

Assessing the individual's learning needs, abilities, preferences, and readiness to learn will help staff determine the best approaches. With pediatric patients, of course, pain management education is primarily geared toward the parents, whether it addresses techniques or assessment skills.

Written materials should accompany verbal instruction to reinforce the message. Written materials include booklets, brochures, instruction sheets, fact sheets, pocket-size cards, and a list of resources for additional pain management information. (See Appendix B for APS List of Resources for Pain Patients 85) The AHRQ has published patient-focused pamphlets for acute pain, cancer pain, and pain in children.

Audio and videotapes can also be helpful teaching tools. If they are left with the individual following an education session, the individual can listen to them more than once to reinforce the message. A program made for the organization's education channel can be viewed repeatedly also. If developed in-house, these materials will probably require the approval of various committees before they are distributed. Video or audio programs can address topics such as medication options, nonpharmacologic interventions, the importance of reporting pain, how to use pain intensity scales, myths of addiction, and the organization's pain management approach, to name a few.

Additionally, satisfaction surveys can help organizations assess individuals' perspectives on pain management. This type of survey can be conducted during pain rounds or during weekly interviews with specific individuals. As an alternative, staff can ask individuals to fill out satisfaction questionnaires, or they can conduct phone surveys following care. Individuals could be asked if they had any pain during their admission. If the answer is yes, they should be asked if they are satisfied with how the physicians and nurses treated their pain.[55] Armed with the results of such surveys, organizations can develop or procure education materials that address the concerns of their population.

Pain questionnaires are another tool. They can be used to help identify individual beliefs and attitudes about pain. These surveys elicit information from individuals about the site and causes of their pain, its effect on their daily function, and their fears of addiction, tolerance, and side effects. Questionnaires can include the Patient Pain Questionnaire, the Wisconsin Brief Pain Inventory, the Brief Symptom Index, the Memorial Symptom Assessment Scale, the Pain Management Index, the Beck Depression Inventory, the Barriers Questionnaire, and the McGill Pain Questionnaire, the last two of which have shortened versions.

Staff cannot assume that all individuals will grasp everything that is taught or be able to raise vital questions during discussions.[71] Therefore, telephone follow up may help the organization ensure that individuals have accurate information and evaluate the efficacy of its education efforts. Another method for ensuring that all important topics have been addressed is to add protocols or checklists to charts and use them to check individual understanding.

Educational efforts can be undertaken by various areas within an organization, and can take various forms. *The Comprehensive Accreditation Manual for Hospitals: The Official Handbook (CAMH)* offers the following to illustrate one approach to implementation of the education standard:

> On reviewing its computer-generated patient information about pain medication, the pharmacy staff might note that the material on opioids does not provide a balanced and accurate reflection of the incidence and severity of possible side effects and cautions for use. The staff could then form a committee to revise these materials, share the revisions with other pharmacies in its system, and forward them to the software developer to include in the next revision of the educational materials for patients.

Chapter 6:

CONTINUUM OF CARE

Health care organizations are responsible for providing adequate information and identifying an appropriate level of follow up health care once individuals served are referred, discharged, or transferred. The Joint Commission standard on continuum of care is this: "The discharge process provides for continuing care based on the individual's assessed needs at the time of discharge." The intent of this Joint Commission standard is that the health care organization not only identifies the individual's continuing needs but arranges for services to meet them and provides relevant information about treatment. For example, when an individual is transferred to another health care organization for pain treatment, information about what has and has not been useful is included in the transfer summary notes.

Categories of individual needs to be considered at discharge include physical; emotional; symptom management, which includes pain; housekeeping; transportation; and social. Discharge planning involves the individual, the family, the practitioner primarily responsible for the individual, nursing and social work professionals, and other appropriate staff. Staff members are responsible for helping the individual and family adapt to the plan of care, which may include postdischarge pain management instructions and follow up.

Chapter 7:

IMPROVING ORGANIZATION PERFORMANCE

To comply with Joint Commission standards, all health care organizations collect data to monitor their performance. Based on its mission, the scope of care, the services provided, and the populations served, every health care organization must choose which processes and outcomes (and thus types of data) are important to monitor. Also, organizations must determine the detail and frequency of data collection appropriate for monitoring ongoing performance. When possible, data collection is incorporated into day-to-day activities rather than performed as a separate activity.

Although organizations have discretion as to what they will measure, they are required to collect data about the needs, expectations, and satisfaction of individuals and organizations they serve. Feedback from individuals and their family members can give an organization insight about process design and functioning. Thus, the organization should ask individuals about their needs and expectations; their perceptions of how well the organization meets these needs and expectations; and how it can improve. The organization can receive input from these groups in a number of ways, including satisfaction surveys, regularly scheduled meetings, and focus groups.

Because pain management covers a vast array of individual needs, many opportunities exist for the organization to measure, and ultimately improve, its performance. The standards offer a list of possible areas for data collection, including the appropriateness and effectiveness of the organization's pain management program. Performance improvement activities are reviewed during the Joint Commission survey process. Performance improvement and the survey are addressed in the following sections.

Performance Improvement Activities
Organizations might measure any of the following:

- Regarding individuals' experience of opioid side effects, knowledge about pain relief, or satisfaction with treatment. Measures focusing on satisfaction could set a goal of 100% compliance for the following events: individuals receiving information on the importance of pain management or individuals reporting satisfaction scores in the 5 to 6 range, 6 being "very satisfied."[59]

- Regarding provider practice patterns of opioid choice, route, and amount; or pain assessment activities, plan of care, and intervention-documentation behavior. More specific measures could include the number or percentage of times that nonpharmacological pain interventions are used, that self-report pain scales are used, that self-administered or regularly scheduled dosing (as opposed to PRN) is used, or that pain reassessment is performed.[34]

The Joint Commission's cycle for improving performance can be applied to a pain management program. For example, an organization may *design* a process for "recognition and treatment of pain." With this in mind, it could revise its nursing documentation to include a space for recording pain intensity/relief measures, identify as a targeted outcome that "nurses screen and record individuals' pain intensity and relief," and set a 90% adherence rate as its goal.[32] It would then *monitor* the staff's performance by collecting documentation data from the clinical records. Is the staff meeting the 90% goal? If not, the organization must *analyze* the data and the process to discover why the goal is not being met and to implement changes. Finally, when the 90% goal is reached, the organization can *improve* by setting a higher goal or focusing on a new performance measure.

Plan and design. The implementation of any new process or the redesign of an existing process should take organizational goals into account. In implementing a pain management program, for example, an organization's goals might be to increase (1) the use of self-report pain scales, (2) the use of self-administered or regularly scheduled dosing (as opposed to PRN), and (3) the frequency of pain assessment. Other goals might be that individuals receive information on the importance of pain management or that no individual waits more than a certain number of minutes for pain medication. Once the goals are clear, the organization develops processes that will help them meet these goals.

Monitor performance through data collection. Data on pain management can be collected from all units and for all shifts to gain a baseline measure of how effectively these new processes are being implemented or, more specifically, how effectively pain is being managed in the organization. Data on all such measures can be collected by conducting interviews and surveys with staff and patients, residents, and clients, and by auditing charts. Outcome data can be collected on specific populations, such as those undergoing certain targeted procedures or those with particular conditions.[33]

Aggregate and analyze data. Once data have been collected, performance improvement tools and techniques such as control charts, flowcharts, cause and effect diagrams, Pareto charts, and root cause analysis can be used to detect and understand the weaknesses of the system: why, for example, pain is not being assessed regularly or why staff lacks knowledge regarding dosing or drug conversion.

Improve. After an organization has analyzed its performance—by pinpointing, for example, how often individuals' pain levels are reassessed, and by whom, or how knowledgeable individuals are about their pain medication—the organization can seek viable ways to *improve* its pain management processes. For example, it could determine appropriate reassessment intervals and set goals for more effective means of educating individuals about their pain management plan.

ORYX Requirements

Depending on an organization's population(s) and services, it may have a variety of viable processes to measure that relate to pain management. Among them are the percentage of nurses and/or physicians screening and recording individuals' pain intensity and relief; the percentage of nurses conducting reassessments; the percentage of staff agreement with preferred answers to a standardized knowledge and attitude assessment tool following educational efforts; the number or percentage of individuals who receive pain management education; the number or percentage of clinical charts that include pain scales; and the number or percentage of individuals who are "very satisfied" with pain management.

Using data on discharge planning, for example, hospitals may find measures to meet its ORYX requirements, the Joint Commission's initiative to integrate performance measures into the accreditation process. The Joint Commission considers the ORYX requirements the next evolution in accreditation that will be implemented over the next several years. Briefly, currently accredited hospitals, long term care organizations, behavioral health care organizations, and home care agencies are required to enroll in at least one performance measurement system chosen from a list of approved systems published by the Joint Commission. Using their chosen system(s), organizations have measures that relate to their respective populations. These accredited organizations are now expected to submit organization- and system-level data for these measures to the Joint Commission over a specified period. Although a number of performance measurement systems have Joint Commission-accepted pain management measures, there is no requirement (either now or planned for the future) for accredited organizations to select one or more pain management measures to report to the Joint Commission as part of the ORYX initiative. New performance measurement expectations are set forth in the chapter entitled "Accreditation Participation Requirements" in each program's *Comprehensive Accreditation Manual*. In addition, the Joint Commission's Web site at www.jcaho.org has the most current information on the ORYX requirements.

Chapter 8:

PAIN ASSESSMENT AND MANAGEMENT IN THE SURVEY

Through the survey process, the Joint Commission will collect information on which new standards are problematic and what types of problems organizations are having with implementation. The review of the pain management standards will not add a separate or new component to the survey process. Rather, surveyors will focus their review as they always have, with the added element of how the organization addresses pain management. Consequently, they may add questions to the existing survey processes and/or review documents related to pain management. In the care interview process, for example, in addition to the typical survey question "What is your assessment process?" the surveyor may also ask, "What is your assessment process for pain?"

In general, key assessment activities that relate to pain management include the following:

Document review. After the opening conference and performance measurement interview, the team reviews documents that will orient surveyors to how the health care organization addresses important functions. These documents focus on the organization's performance. They include committee minutes, reports of measurement and assessment activities, and reports to medical staff, health care organization commit-

tees, and the governing body. Certain bylaws, planning documents, and other evidence of performance will also be included. For pain management, surveyors may review minutes of a meeting at which a team developed a pain management care pathway or other approach. They may then ask to see policies and procedures, clinical practice guidelines, or protocols the organization uses.

Interviews with organization leaders. The leadership interview takes place early in the survey, after the document review and before visits to care settings. It addresses the collaboration of senior leaders in planning, designing, implementing, and improving care services. A question regarding how the organization demonstrates its commitment to pain management may be asked of this group. Other interviews with organization leaders address specific roles of administration, medical staff and nursing leaders, and departmental directors in addressing pain management issues. These other interviews take place later in the survey to allow surveyors to approach the interviews with greater knowledge of the organization's performance.

Visits to care settings. The team may spend as much as half its time visiting places where individuals receive care and services to assess performance in these settings. These visits address how the organization's functions perform together in the care process. Surveyors will also address how planning and design processes for pain management have been implemented and improved.

Function interviews. These interviews gather a multidisciplinary group who have important responsibilities related to pain management. They follow up on issues identified in the document review and reflect observations made by surveyors in visits to care settings. The interviews will be conducted by one or more surveyors.

Each interview includes

- introduction of surveyor(s) to the group gathered for the interview;

- introduction of participants and their role in performing the function;

- brief statement of the purpose of the interview and its relationship to other survey activities;

- interview of participants addressing issues related to the function and how the function has been planned, designed, implemented, measured, assessed, and, as appropriate, improved; and

- concluding comments.

The interviews also

- address issues identified by all surveyors from observations made before the interview;

- address issues raised during the document review session, leadership interview, and visits to care settings; and

- include any appropriate comments of an educational or helpful nature as long as they

do not interfere with the interview's evaluative purpose.

Function interviews include, for example, the

- ethics interview;

- continuum of care interview;

- infection control interview;

- information management interview;

- human resources interview;

- medical staff credentials interview;

- patient care interview;

- performance improvement team interview(s); and

- performance improvement coordinating group interview.

Other assessment activities. Certain survey activities involve staff with specific responsibilities related to the pain management standards, for example, the

- admitting services visit;

- pharmacy services visit; and

- medical record interview.

Feedback sessions. Final scores for compliance are not tallied until all care settings have been visited and all other assessment interviews and activities have been conducted. However, surveyors will communicate their observations at daily briefings and during a medical staff conference luncheon if such a luncheon is requested. At the leadership exit conference, complete survey findings and a preliminary written report and accreditation decision will be discussed with staff, at the discretion of the chief executive officer.

Chapter 9:

CASE STUDIES

Hospital Case Study: *Abbott Northwestern Hospital and the Virginia Piper Cancer Institute*

The Pain Project, a joint clinical QI initiative of Abbott Northwestern Hospital and the Virginia Piper Cancer Institute, was established in 1995 to improve the management of pain for all patients hospitalized for surgery or cancer.

What had to be improved at the 597-bed tertiary care Minneapolis-based institution? Survey data revealed that patients who had open heart surgery had inadequate pain management, 83% of patients who had a microdiscectomy had postoperative pain, meperidine was widely prescribed, and there was inconsistent documentation with five pain charting forms used throughout the organization, recalls Paula Sallmen, RN, BA, OCN, clinical program director.

The three-year long project was spearheaded by a multidisciplinary panel composed of physicians, nurses, pharmacists, a clinical researcher, and clergy. The goal was to improve pain management through the widespread dissemination and use of well-documented, accepted, and evidence-based research and guidelines, including the AHQR acute and cancer pain management guidelines. (See Figure 9.1).

The Pain Project team, which met monthly, developed project principles to provide philosophical guidance. For example, the patient-focused emphasis encouraged all clinicians to work together, thus diluting issues of territory. The evidence-based principle emphasized scientific knowledge over personal preference and habit.

After developing an implementation strategies flow chart to determine how the agreed-upon interventions would be operationalized, the team selected patient populations to monitor as part of the project. Patient population selections were based on the following rationale:

- Pain is a patient-reported problem;

- Providers voiced a need for improved pain management;

- Volume of patients affected;

- Amount of analgesics used;

- Maturity of the interdisciplinary governance structure within the patient care unit; and

- Feasibility or timing of other competitive initiatives.

Figure 9.1 Objectives of Clinical PI Project

The purpose of the clinical improvement project is to prevent or manage pain for all patients hospitalized for surgery or cancer through education and system changes. Project objectives are presented here with project actions, outcomes, and outcome measures.

1. Educate patients about pain management so they can receive prompt evaluation and effective treatment.
   Action: Every patient will receive the Patient Fact Sheet or AHCPR pamphlet and actively participate in pain assessment and management.
   Outcome: Patient knowledge about pain will increase.
   Measure: Patient Pain Interview (Ferrell, 1995b.)

2. Increase research-based pain management behavior by physicians, nurses and pharmacists.
   Action: Provide physicians, nurses and pharmacists with information on the AHCPR Guidelines. Modify physician orders to reflect Guidelines. Improve written pain plans of care.
   Outcome: Provider pain management knowledge increases. Appropriate drugs, doses, route and schedule are ordered and administered. Complementary therapies are used. Complete assessments of pain are documented and therapy approximates assessment. A pain management plan of care is evident for each patient. Medication side effects are assessed, prevented and managed.
   Measure: Knowledge and Attitude Survey (Ferrell, 1995c); Pain Chart Audit (Ferrell, 1995a.)

3. Reduce the incidence and severity of surgical and cancer related pain, and increase patient satisfaction with pain management.
   Action: Assessment, prevention and intervention for pain conducted according to the Guidelines.
   Outcome: Patient's perceived pain intensity will decrease. Patient satisfaction with pain management will be higher.
   Measure: Patient Pain Interview (Ferrell, 1995b.)

4. Ensure an ongoing, institutional commitment and accountability for pain management.
   Actions: Include pain management in quality management plans. Work with quality management to develop a standard for patient pain and comfort. Use pain management indicator to support consistent and prompt assessment, diagnosis, intervention and documentation relative to patient pain management.
   Outcome: A retrievable and useful indicator of patient pain management.
   Measure: Evidence of indicator use to advance the pain plan of care.

Source: Abbott Northwestern Hospital and the Virginia Piper Cancer Institute, Minneapolis, MN. Used with permission.

An opinion leader and change agent were chosen for each patient population and physician group to champion the pain initiative.

A pain management patient care improvement report summarized project activity for each patient care unit. Implementation strategies and clinical products, outcomes, feedback, present and future work, and contacts were included in this packet. The report was updated and distributed after each implementation stage.

Education was the cornerstone of the Pain Project, says Sallmen. Each clinician was viewed as accountable for the assessment, intervention, and outcomes of pain management.

An eight-hour formal classroom education program based on pain management principles was provided for all nurses and pharmacists. Faculty from across disciplines were involved in the program that included all aspects of a holistic, total person approach to pain management. Participants received a Pain Manual that addressed objectives of the pain education program, anatomy and physiology of pain, case presentation, pain management assessment, pharmacologic therapy, spiritual considerations, research and data components, nonpharmacologic strategy, case discussion, and the institutional pain standard. Currently, an interactive CD-ROM is being developed to educate new staff.

The hospital leaders' support was evident by their willingness to finance the time required for staff to attend classes, which were offered regularly for the project's duration. Managers allowed for flexible scheduling to ensure attendance by hospital staff members.

Given their time constraints, physician education was formatted differently. Pain management updates were consistently and regularly provided at physician meetings. For example, formal presentations were made at joint practice councils, department meetings, and medical staff meetings. They included discussion of the project principles, follow-up data, and appropriate content for preprinted physician orders. Academic detailing techniques were used to assist in gaining physician buy-in and to facilitate practice change.

The panel developed an institutional pain standard that was approved by the hospital's patient care committee. (See Figure 9.2 for Standards of Pain Management for Patients at Abbott Northwestern Hospital.) The standard, based on the AHQR guidelines and other literature, demonstrates the organization's ongoing commitment to research-based pain management.

Standing orders were implemented for every surgical and oncology patient population. The preprinted physician orders address assessment, medication type, dosing, side effect prevention, and discontinuation of therapy. The new orders, which replaced previous ones, are flexible enough to allow for variation in patient and physician preferences. Additionally, algorithms were developed that address continuous infusion for morphine or hydromorphone, conversion from continuous infusion to oral administration, management of painful bone metastases, and management of neuropathic pain. Also, pain rating scales were made consistent across hospital care units. However, each clinical area decided about the placement of scales on the unit (such as posted on pocket-size laminated card, laminated to the back of the patient clipboard, or hung at the patient's bedside).

Documentation revisions assisted clinicians in complying with the new approach. For example, a pain management plan prompted them to record daily outcomes, pharmacologic treatments, and nonpharmacologic interventions. A revised flowsheet enabled trending of patterns in

Figure 9.2 Standards of Pain Management: for Patients

Goal
All patients will receive the best level of pain control that can safely be provided.

Scope
These standards apply to patients with acute and/or cancer-related pain. Management of chronic nonmalignant pain is beyond the scope of these standards and may require additional evaluations and different interventions.

Standards of care for pain management:

Assessment

A. All patients will be assessed for pain upon admission.
B. When pain is an identified problem, individualized pain management goals will be established and regular assessments will take place until the problem is resolved.
C. Pain assessment includes location and intensity; but in most cases should include other dimensions such as psychosocial and spiritual distress.
D. Chemically dependent patients may require additional assessment, closer monitoring and more patient, family and health care provider education; but the goals and the treatment elements are the same as for the nonchemically dependent patient.

Intervention

A. If pain is rated > 4/10 or is unacceptable to the patient, there will be an intervention to reduce the pain.
B. If pain is not improving after 24 hours, additional measures should be taken unless reasons for waiting longer are documented.
C. Adverse effects of treatment will be anticipated and monitored in a timely manner.
D. Patients and their families will receive timely education about pain relief.
E. Complementary therapies will be available and offered when appropriate.
F. Unless pain is occurring only occasionally, scheduled analgesics are indicated with additional medication available on demand for breakthrough pain.
G. Oral and intravenous administration of analgesics are preferred over intramuscular administration.
H. Opioids are considered to be the analgesics of choice for moderate to severe pain.
I. Meperidine is generally not preferred for pain management; if used it should not be administered for more than four consecutive days due to accumulation of toxic metabolites.
J. Suitable conversions should be made when switching opioid analgesics or their route of administration.
K. Non steroidal anti-inflammatory agents are beneficial but need to be administered judiciously considering the risk of adverse effects. Ketoroiac (both parenteral and oral) should not be administered for longer than five consecutive days.
L. If pain is likely to persist beyond the hospitalization, a plan for outpatient pain management should be instituted.

Documentation

A. The initial pain assessment should be documented in the hospital chart.
B. Subsequent assessments should be readily accessible and become part of the permanent record.
C. Standardized forms adopted by Abbott Northwestern Hospital should be used for reporting pain assessments and analgesic monitoring.
D. Progress notes should clearly delineate the plan and rational for pain treatment.

Institutional Responsibility
Abbott Northwestern Hospital will continue to monitor the way pain is managed through the Quality Management Department and Continuous Quality Improvement programs.

Source: Abbott Northwestern Hospital and the Virginia Piper Cancer Institute, Minneapolis, MN. Used with permission.

assessment, intervention, and response to therapy over time.

Other clinical products used to assist and support providers in implementing the AHQR guidelines include the following:

- Copies of AHQR acute and cancer pain management guidelines;

- Pain assessment scales, including a 0 to 10 pain intensity scale reference in color, a faces scale, a descriptor scale, and a numeric pain scale; and

- Fact sheets, located at point-of-care, that summarized key AHQR pain management principles.

Like clinicians, patients were given a variety of educational pieces. The panel developed a fact sheet that defines pain and summarizes treatment as well as emphasizes and encourages patient participation in pain management. Educational efforts also attempt to correct patients' misconceptions about pain and its management. A laminated card with pain assessment scales was developed to assist patients in describing their pain. AHQR patient-focused pamphlets provide information about treatment goals, pain control methods and plans, relaxation techniques, numeric pain intensity ratings, and medications.

Outcomes measured before and after the Pain Project interventions were implemented include

- patient pain experience (intensity, function, opioid side effects, knowledge, and satisfaction);

- clinician practice patterns (opioid choice, route, and dose; assessment, plan of care, and intervention documentation behavior; and knowledge); and

- system factors (LOS and drug costs).

Data were collected via interview, questionnaire, and chart audit. Provider knowledge and attitudes were measured by the Knowledge and Attitude Survey Regarding Pain and practice patterns were measured using the Pain Chart Audit. Outcomes data were collected for oncology patients with pain and for patients undergoing coronary artery bypass graft, hysterectomy, total joint or knee replacement, cesarean section, craniotomy, and laminectomy surgery.

As a result of the Pain Project, the following pain management improvements have been documented:

- Patient satisfaction increased between 5% and 19% across populations;

- Pain intensity ratings improved slightly;

- Ambulation improved;

- Opioid-related side effects did not increase, and the number of patients' reporting moderate or severe nausea decreased by 22%;

- Documentation of pain plans of care increased by an average of 40%;

- Morphine use increased and meperidine use decreased;

- IM opioid administration was virtually eliminated;

- PCA and epidural pain management were used more frequently; and

- Preemptive pain management was strengthened.

Long Term Care Case Study:
Brandywine Nursing Home

In 1997, Brandywine Nursing Home in Westchester County, New York, decided to make pain management the focus of a quality assurance (QA) project. Two residents with very complicated pain problems were actually the impetus behind the project, explains Jill Loeb, RN, BSN, QA coordinator and pain management specialist at the 131-bed LTC facility. When Loeb investigated the circumstances of both residents after learning about them in an interdisciplinary care plan meeting, she realized that the pain relief they had been getting was ineffective and inconsistently documented.

Next, a chart review for all residents was conducted to see how many residents were getting pain medication, and how staff were assessing and documenting the effectiveness of treatment. Then Loeb interviewed the majority of residents, that is, all who were capable of participating. She asked what pain medication they were taking, whether it was working, was the pain interfering with their ADLs, and whether they were able to enjoy their social activities. The data revealed that 55% of the LTC's residents were receiving some form of medication to treat pain. However, 25% of those did not have well controlled pain. "At that point we realized that we needed some mechanism in place to identify residents who needed pain control," says Loeb. "We also needed a consistent means for the assessment, documentation, and evaluation of interventions."

An interdisciplinary pain management committee was formed. It consisted of representatives from nursing, medicine, pharmacy, social work, physical therapy, occupational therapy, dietary, and recreation. The team agreed to first focus on the assessment process. As part of an extensive literature search, Loeb collected multiple examples of assessment tools. Unable to find one tool appropriate for Brandywine residents, she used pieces from several tools to design one most suited for the facility. For example, she wanted to include a question about ADLs and rehabilitation. "We have a lot of people who are on restorative physical or occupational therapy, and one of the things I was looking at is whether pain was interfering with their performance," she says. An additional tool was developed for residents who are unable to self-report. (See Figure 9.3 for Assessment Tool for Residents Unable to Self Report.)

As part of the new pain assessment process, a nurse evaluates all new admissions and readmissions, as well as residents who have a change of status or at a minimum of quarterly. The assessment includes

- interviewing the resident using the pain assessment tool (including filling out the diagram to show where the pain is);

- listing pain management interventions in use;

- teaching/reinforcing the use of the pain rating scale;

- obtaining a qualitative description (in the resident's own words);

- documenting aggravating and alleviating factors; and

- discussing the effect of pain on the resident's quality of life and ADLs.

For residents unable to answer the assessment questions, for example, those who are severely cognitively impaired or comatose, the assessment process includes

- evaluating the resident's diagnosis and physical status for potentially painful conditions;

Figure 9.3 Brandywine Nursing Home Pain Assessment Tool for Residents Unable to Self Report

RESIDENT _____ UNIT/RM # _____

1) Diagnosis (pathology) which predisposes resident to pain: _____
_____
_____

2) Potentially painful treatment / procedure: _____
_____
_____

3) Family assessment (0-10): _____
comments: _____

4) Licensed Nurse assessment: (0-10): _____
comments: _____

5) Behaviors exhibited that may be indicative of pain: (CRYING, GROOMING, GRIMACING)
_____
_____

Additional Comments: _____
_____
_____

Disposition:
_____ No evidence of pain (will reassess as needed)

_____ Mild, occasional & well controlled pain
_____ Pain Management Program

Nurse's signature: _____ Date: _____

Source: Brandywine Nursing Home, Westchester County, NY. Used with permission.

- listing painful or potentially painful treatments/procedures the resident is receiving;

- interviewing family members or significant others regarding their perception of the resident's pain or discomfort;

- interviewing primary caregivers regarding their assessments of the resident's pain or discomfort; and

- documenting behaviors exhibited by the resident that may be indicative of pain.

In general, the 0 to 10 Numeric Pain Intensity Scale is preferred for assessment. For residents who are unable to use this scale, verbal descriptor scales can be used. Loeb discourages the use of a pain faces scale as she found many of the residents and their families view it as condescending.

Staff then arrives at a disposition, which helps them tailor a pain care plan, for each resident. For example, the first disposition says, "No evidence of pain." These residents neither require nor receive pain interventions. However, they will be reassessed as needed. The second category is for those experiencing "mild, occasional, and well controlled pain." These residents' care plans typically will include a prescription for non-opioid analgesics as well as nonpharmacologic interventions, such as guided imagery, and require follow-up and monitoring. The third disposition for those who have "objectively or subjectively demonstrated ineffective pain control" are placed in the Pain Management Program. The care plan for these residents will most often include both pharmacologic interventions, ranging from opioids to adjuvant analgesics, and nonpharmacologic strategies, including physical therapy, relaxation techniques, and stress management.

In addition to the assessment tool, the committee developed a flowsheet for staff to document the effectiveness of the pain management regimen on every shift. The initial flowsheet was very complicated, but through subsequent revisions was simplified. (See Figure 9.4 for Pain Relief Flow Sheet.) One item added was the question, "Is pain relief acceptable to the resident?" "We added that right onto the flowsheet because that's why we're doing it," explains Loeb. "It's sort of instant QA." The flowsheet calls for

- listing all medications being used for pain treatment;

- assessing the resident at a minimum of once per shift regarding the presence of pain until satisfactory relief is achieved;

- reassessing the resident one hour after medicating or performing intervention; and

- assessing the presence of medication side effects.

The flowsheet is initiated as soon as a resident is placed in the program and is continued until effective pain relief is achieved and maintained over time.

A care plan guide was developed to assist in individualizing treatment plans. It includes a problem statement, for example, "The resident has osteoarthritis and experiences knee pain, rated between a 3 and 4, that increases with weight bearing activities." A list of interventions may include "acetaminophen, physical therapy, and guided imagery," with a note like, "Resident verbalizes satisfactory pain relief with acetaminophen." The goal may read, "Resident wants to be able to get into and out of bed without discomfort." Loeb says she prefers using functional goals because they focus on what the resident actually does, and therefore are more relevant to the patient. "They're measurable and you can develop a care plan to meet a functional goal utilizing a multidisciplinary approach. It helps us to take pain relief beyond just giving a

Figure 9.4 Brandywine Nursing Home Pain Relief Flow Sheet

Resident _____

Unit/Rm _____

Date _____

Current Medications for Pain: (Please note changes in meds and the date of the change) _____

_____

_____

Date _____

Time _____

_____ Pain Rating at time of medication admin (0-10) mild/moderate/severe

_____ Pain Rating 1 hour after med given (0-10) mild/moderate/severe

Is pain relief acceptable to resident? Yes or No

Comments (Side Effects) (obj observations) _____

Initial _____

Source: Brandywine Nursing Home, Westchester County, NY. Used with permission.

pill," she explains. All disciplines involved in pain management are documented on the care plan, which include ongoing pain assessments and intervention evaluations. The consultant pharmacist is a crucial resource in establishing and evaluating pharmacological interventions. There are also periodic reviews by the pharmacy consultant to monitor the medication regime and to make appropriate recommendations for approved pain management. Narrative notes are written in the care plan at least monthly for residents in the Pain Management Program and, at a minimum, quarterly for all other residents. Pain management care plans are reviewed quarterly with the residents. Loeb is responsible for reviewing all pain assessments and documentation. In addition, the committee incorporated pain management for the first time into the nursing policy and procedure manual.

An important component of Brandywine's pain management initiative is staff education. To that end, staff is educated about addiction, physical dependence, and tolerance as well as misconceptions surrounding pain and its treatment. All staff is taught to look for nonverbal pain cues, including grimacing, moaning, or rubbing a body part. Additionally, they are sensitized to other less obvious cues of behavior changes, such as depression, restlessness, agitation, withdrawal, loss of appetite, or a decline in performance of ADLs. This information is included in orientation for all new staff, as well as in in service programs conducted twice annually. Pain management education has also been incorporated into in-services on residents' rights. Consequently, it carries more weight because it is taught as a mandated class, says Loeb.

But staff education reaches beyond nursing, she notes. As part of their orientation, all new maintenance, housekeeping, and dietary staff are taught to look for nonverbal cues of pain. Often times, residents don't want to bother the nurses, she says. But maintenance personnel will see the patient rubbing his or her neck, or the resident will complain to the housekeeping staff of pain. "We get some of our best referrals from them because we key everyone into looking for pain, and not just waiting for residents to verbalize it," notes Loeb.

Resident education starts on the day of admission, says Loeb, who interviews and assesses all new residents. They are taught how to report pain and use pain rating scales as well as why PRN medications are necessary to treat pain before it becomes severe. The concept that pain is not a normal part of aging is stressed, she says. Residents are encouraged to report pain to keep it under control. They must be assured that their reports of pain will be accepted and acted upon, Loeb notes. Because residents do not necessarily have pain upon admission, those without pain are reassessed periodically or as needed. When pain becomes an issue, then the family is typically notified, as well. Residents also receive a booklet that includes an explanation of the facility's pain management program, a definition of pain and pain management, and a list of resident responsibilities. The latter recommends the following:

• Report pain to the nursing staff when it occurs;

• Report increases in pain intensity to the nursing staff;

• Be a part of the interdisciplinary team working towards managing your pain; and

• Verbalize your questions or concerns regarding your pain, pain medications, or pain management regime, to members of the "pain management team."

The committee developed a QA audit tool to determine the effectiveness of the pain management initiative. Three to four residents per unit are chosen randomly to be interviewed every couple of months. Results show a significant decrease in pain ratings with a correlation to increased participation of ADLs. In addition, a "Quality of Life" survey conducted through the Recreation Department and Social Services biannually to determine resident satisfaction includes questions about pain management. Loeb prefers using the functional goals listed in the care plan to determine the program's success. For example, one resident's goal was to sleep through the night uninterrupted by pain. There is documented evidence that she is doing so. Another resident with arthritis pain wanted to be able to resume her needlework, which she is now doing.

Overall, residents report an improved ability to sleep, increased independence in ADLs, greater participation in recreational activities, and general heightened feelings of well-being and control over their health and lives, notes Loeb. Their families talk about the return of the person they know and love, and express increased peace of mind and the ability to enjoy quality time together.

Home Care Case Study: *University of Wisconsin Hospital and Clinics Home Health Agency*

With an increasing number of patients who have pain issues being discharged into the University of Wisconsin Hospital and Clinics Home Health Agency's care, the Madison-based organization set out to improve pain management outcomes.

Backed by administrative support and funding, the agency hired two nurse consultants who had worked with its affiliated hospital to establish the Wisconsin Cancer Pain Initiative. An interdisciplinary workgroup was formed. It was composed of the nurse consultants, pharmacy staff, a physical therapist, a clinical applications nurse, and a primary nurse.

The agency's objectives were to

- demonstrate institutional commitment to managing pain;

- continue quality pain management into the home care and community settings;

- implement the PI process in pain management;

- make pain a visible issue within the organization; and

- improve pain management practice patterns.

The first step was to study the agency's current pain management practices and documentation patterns. In May 1994, the workgroup conducted random chart audits. The medical record review revealed inconsistencies in documentation and a lack of focus on pain as an issue. "We realized that our documentation system did not prompt nurses to focus on pain as a problem," recalls Barbara Liegel, director of the home health agency that averages 200 patients on service and conducts between 1300 and 1400 visits a month. Although pain was mentioned in 19 of the 25 records reviewed, it was not documented with any systematic frequency. In fact, pain issues were documented less than one time per week, with very few descriptors of pain character or intensity.

Consequently, the first improvement focused on establishing and implementing a standard of practice to determine when pain is to be followed as a patient problem. (See Figure 9.5 for UWHC Standard of Practice.) To that end, the workgroup revised the Admission Assessment Form to prompt nurses to assess the presence or absence of pain in each patient. The 0 to 10 Numeric Pain Intensity Scale and the Pain Faces Scale were agreed upon by the interdisciplinary group. They are the same scales used in the hospital and it was thought that their use would promote continuity of care, says Liegel. If the patient is experiencing pain, then the nurse also completes a newly created Pain Assessment Form. This form guides the nurse in obtaining a comprehensive description of the pain, including intensity, location, quality, aggravating and alleviating factors, and patient concerns and goals. In addition, the workgroup developed and implemented a Pain Management Flow Sheet for the documentation of interventions.

A pain resource nurse in home health was added to the staff. The pain resource nurse provides pain management education and consultation to other staff nurses.

Another objective was to provide staff education. The nurse consultants, along with pharmacy staff from the Wisconsin Cancer Pain Initiative, conducted a series of in-services for the staff. Topics included pain transmission, assessment, and common misconceptions; nonparenteral administration of opioids; opioid dose conversion and titration; use of non-opioid medications and

Figure 9.5 University of Wisconsin Hospital and Clinics Home Health Agency: Standard of Practice

1. Patients will be informed verbally at the time of their initial evaluation, and in an electronic or printed format, that effective pain relief is an important part of their treatment, that their report of unrelieved pain is essential, and that staff will respond quickly to patients' reports of pain.

2. On initial evaluation and as part of regular and routine assessments, all patients will be asked about the presence and intensity of pain. The initial assessment will involve a complete history and physical exam including the patient's self report of pain intensity (using numeric rating scale when possible), pain quality, location, temporal characteristics, aggravating and alleviating factors, effects of pain on function and quality of life, and response to past interventions. Ongoing assessment is essential. The degree of pain relief should be determined after pain treatment once sufficient time has elapsed to reach peak effect.

3. Each patient will have a clearly articulated goal for pain relief. The goal should be stated as a point on the pain intensity scale which the patient understands will result in a dose adjustment or other intervention. In addition to an identified pain intensity rating, the goal may be articulated in relation to other criteria such as functional-status or quality of life.

4. Pain that persists above the pain relief goal will trigger an interdisciplinary review of the plan of care and modification in treatment.

The Standard is Accomplished Through:

AHCPR patient guide principles of acute pain management are summarized in all written pre-op patient education packets.

Copies of the AHCPR patient guide on cancer pain is available in all oncology patient care areas.

Service standards address promise of comfort, and are posted in all clinic and inpatient rooms.

Health Fact for You "What Everyone Should Know about Pain Management" is available in all settings.

Integration of pain assessment standard in documentation policy (ongoing assessment parameters), nursing flow-sheets, and all critical pathways.

Documentation of the patient's pain relief goal is completed in the outcome section of all critical pathways or outpatient plan of care.

For persistent pain above the identified goal (> 5 two consecutive assessments in a 4 hour period at rest, or over a 24 hour period with activity, or if the patient is not satisfied with pain relief) the narrative summary addresses the pain management plan and the unrelieved pain algorithm is followed (see pg 7).

Regardless of the setting (clinic, inpatient unit, ICU, home health), or patient population (pediatric, adult, geriatric), unrelieved pain is communicated by the RN through a regular reporting mechanism to other caregivers, and interventions are planned, coordinated, and carried out.

Source: University of Wisconsin Hospital and Clinics Home Health Agency, Madison, WI. Used with permission.

the treatment of neuropathic pain; invasive therapies and nonpharmacologic interventions; and myths that inhibit the expression and relief of pain. In-services were conducted three to four times annually and offered at two different times to make it easier for all staff to attend. A six-part Cancer Pain Management Education program that focused on assessment, basic pain theory, and pharmacologic and nonpharmacologic interventions, was also offered.

A self-directed learning guide was developed to provide staff nurses with a review of the standard of practice for pain management. Also included is the nursing competency for pain management, an algorithm to assess and report unrelieved pain, and a summary of principles of pain management. (See Figure 9.6 for Principles of Pain Management.) The guide comes with a posttest to evaluate the effectiveness of the educational effort. In addition, all nurses receive a copy of the AHQR pain management guidelines and a pocket-size Pain Reference Card. Videotapes by pain management experts are available for view. New staff is given all of this information as part of orientation and is required to spend time with the PRN.

Additionally, the nurse consultants role-modeled pain assessment and intervention by providing telephone support and accompanying agency staff on home visits. During the visits, they would provide consultation to improve pain control and symptom management. In addition, a staff pharmacist was also available to discuss patient-specific issues as needed.

Among the myriad of patient education materials gathered for distribution are the following:

- AHQR's patient guide principles of acute pain management are summarized in all written preoperative patient education packets;

- AHQR's patient guide on cancer pain are available in all oncology patient care areas;

- Service standards stating that all patients' reports of pain will be responded to promptly are posted in all clinic and inpatient rooms; and

- A pamphlet entitled "What Everyone Should Know about Pain Management" is available in all settings.

After the educational interventions were conducted and the tools implemented, the workgroup performed another chart audit. In 1994, baseline data showed that pain was documented three times per record. In 1995, after the educational sessions, role-modeling, and assessment form interventions were implemented, pain was documented 8 times per record, and an assessment form was completed for 8 out of 21 patients upon admission. In 1996, after the standard was set, the flowsheet was implemented, and the role-modeling sessions were repeated, pain assessments were completed for 15 out of 17 patients upon admission, and 12 out of 17 also had a flowsheet.

In 1998, the agency purchased a new computer system, and in 1999 the whole pain management process was being rebuilt on the new system. Concurrently, the agency became a participant in a Robert Wood Johnson Foundation funded initiative aimed at improving pain management practices of 25 local home health agencies. As part of the initiative, an indicator was used to measure documentation. Specifically, it called for documentation of pain to be addressed with every admission, and that an appropriate pain assessment should include a description of the location and character of the pain, and a rating on a recognized, acceptable pain scale. An initial medical record audit revealed that the agency had four weak areas:

Figure 9.6 Principles of Pain Management

The patient's self report is the single most reliable indicator of pain. When possible use a numeric (0-10, 0-5) or descriptive (mild-moderate-severe) pain intensity scale to assess and document pain severity.

Prevention is better than treatment.

Base the initial choice of analgesic on the severity and type of pain: mon-opioids for mild pain (rating 1-4); opioids, often in combination with a non-opioid, for moderate (rating 5-6) to severe (rating 7-10) pain. Neuropathic pain may require an antidepressant or anticonvulsant drug.

Dose to the maximum dose of non-opioid if side effects permit. There is no maximum dose or analgesic ceiling with most opioids. Increase opioid dose until pain relief is achieved or side effects are unmanageable before changing medications.

Administer drugs orally whenever possible. Avoid intramuscular injections.

Administer analgesics "around the clock" rather than pm.

Avoid using multiple opioids or multiple non-opioids (drugs from the same class at the same time) when possible.

Opioids should be titrated by a percentage of the current dose based on intensity of pain
• for mild to moderate pain by 25-50%
• for moderate to severe pain by 50-100%

Anticipate and vigorously treat side effects.

Avoid dosing with meperidine (no more than 48 hours or at doses greater than 600mg/24 hours). Accumulation of toxic metabolite normeperidine (half-life = 12-16 hrs) can lead to CNS excitability and convulsions. Contraindicated in patients with impaired renal function or those receiving MAO inhibitors.

Nonpharmacologic interventions are intended to supplement, not substitute for pharmacologic interventions.

Addiction occurs very rarely in patients who receive opioids for pain control. Drug addiction, when suspected should be investigated and ruled in or out but not implied and 'left hanging' because it interferes with pain management. The hallmarks of addiction include a) compulsive use, b) loss of control, and c) use in spite of harm.

Do not use placebos to determine if the pain is "real."

Assess pain, pain relief, and side effects frequently and adjust the dose accordingly. Change to another drug if side effects are unmanageable.

Source: University of Wisconsin Hospital and Clinics Home Health Agency, Madison, WI. Excerpt from UWHC *Self-Directed Learning Guide: Pain Management.* Copyright 1998 UW Hospital and Clinics Authority Board. Used with permission.

1. Pain character and pain rating on a 0 to 10 numerical scale were not being documented.

2. Staff was not being accountable for pain management as it was not integrated into staff performance evaluation.

3. With the transition to the new computer system, staff was overlooking existing pain documentation standards. Consequently, documentation of pain management goals and outcomes had not been monitored and reported through PI process.

4. The patient Bill of Rights did not inform patients and families about the importance of pain relief.

The agency is currently addressing these areas of improvement in a variety of ways. For example, the results of the initial audit were shared with staff at an in-service in March, 1999. The in-service addressed documentation of pain assessment, intervention, goals, and outcomes. Although the new computer system enables staff to easily document the presence or absence of pain and its location, where exactly to document this information is confusing, says Liegel. Consequently, the fields in the computer system are being rebuilt to facilitate meeting the documentation standard. Documentation of pain management will become the focus of a monthly chart audit, results of which will be shared with staff. In addition, the audit findings and competency achievement will be incorporated into the annual staff performance evaluation. Finally, the Patient Bill of Rights will be reviewed and updated to include information about the importance of pain relief.

A final audit revealed an improvement in how often the documentation indicates the presence of pain, its location and character, as well as the use of a pain scale.

In the future, the workgroup plans to conduct patient surveys to determine the incidence of pain, the effectiveness of the interventions, and patient-related barriers. As an agency certified by the Health Care Financing Administration, it participates in the Outcome and Assessment Information Set (OASIS), an outcomes assessment tool that includes questions upon admission about pain management. The PRN will monitor those responses as well as adherence to the standard of care through periodic medical record reviews. Ongoing staff training and in-service will continue and will expand on the use of electronic and other media.

"Pain will always be a quality indicator or part of the PI process here," says Liegel. "You have to continually evaluate and work to improve the quality of pain management. But it's important to remember that it's a process. You should set a standard and continue to strive for it."

Behavorial Health Care Case Study:
CARITAS Peace Center

Spurred by the ethical debate regarding end-of-life care and the notion of providing compassionate care, the CARITAS Peace Center, a 200-bed behavioral health care facility in Louisville, Kentucky, began assessing how it manages pain for its patients with psychiatric and behavioral problems.

In fact, pain management became the focus of the entire health system Sisters of Charity of Nazareth Health Systems with which the Peace Center was affiliated in 1994. Pain management education became a systemwide goal for the fiscal year 1994-1995, which included a full orientation to methods of pain management for all physicians, nurses, and allied health professionals.

Concurrent with the formation of a corporate pain management committee, CARITAS Health Services, which is composed of the Peace Center, the Pain Management Center, CARITAS Medical Center, a home health agency, and outpatient clinics, established its own committee in 1994. Because pain management was being addressed systemwide, the approximately 21-member committee included representatives from all of the SCN Health System facilities, including individuals from education, nursing, activity therapy, pastoral care, and social services. Each of the SCN Health System facilities had established its own pain management committee to identify issues specific to the site and implement interventions. The items addressed at the various facility committee meetings, which were held monthly, were reported to the corporate committee. As a result, many interventions and tools used to improve pain management at one facility were adopted for use by other ones, notes Andrew Meyer, PhD, who was director of the CARITAS

Health Service's Pain Management Center and served as chair of the CARITAS Pain Management Committee.

The center's committee members determined that education was a priority, beginning with educating themselves about all the relevant issues regarding pain management. To that end, they conducted an extensive literature search, compiling hundreds of journal articles. In addition, they culled information from organizations, such as the American Pain Society and the American Academy of Pain Medicine.

Next, a subcommittee researched appropriate needs assessment tools. The committee administered the Nurses' Knowledge and Attitudes Survey Regarding Pain to determine baseline staff knowledge. The committee not only used the results to provide feedback to staff, but also to develop topics for educational efforts. For example, the feedback showed that while staff was knowledgeable with respect to physiology, they were less familiar with psychosocial and pharmacological interventions, Meyer recalls. Consequently, the committee developed a videotape that discusses the feedback and then elaborates on the use of relaxation techniques, imagery, and biofeedback, among others. The videotape was sent to all of the units to be presented at unit meetings. To date, four videotapes addressing staff attitudes and knowledge have been completed.

Other staff barriers that were revealed were that the clinicians', and in particular the physicians', were reasonably well trained in treating acute pain, but not necessarily as aware of addressing chronic pain states or the interaction between the physical and mental components of pain. In addition, some staff automatically assumed that patients are seeking drugs if they requested more pain medication, says Delores

Gatewood, BSN, RNC, a clinical applications specialist at the Peace Center. Moreover, as a behavioral health facility co-managing patients who have addictions or substance abuse histories with appropriate pain medications is more of an issue than is concern about causing patients to become addicted. This limited knowledge of pain and its mechanisms as well as addiction and substance abuse concerns are common staff barriers as borne out in the medical literature. Consequently, educational efforts stressed the distinction between primary and secondary addiction, which has treatment implications. The former describing patients with a history of drug abuse/addiction prior to the incidence of pain and the latter being patients who, until the current pain episode, had rarely used medications. Terms, such as addiction, psychological dependence versus physical dependence, drug abuse, and pseudoaddiction, were clearly defined in all educational materials.

Committee members agreed that educational efforts should provide general principles of pain education, describe psychological problems that increase pain (fear, isolation, depression, insomnia, anxiety), and identify myths regarding pain (lying about the existence of pain, malingering, is common; visible signs, either psychological or behavioral, accompany pain and can be used to verify its existence and severity; a noncompliant patient probably does not want to feel better).

The committee's educational efforts were rolled out beginning in August 1995. A two-day pain management training program was held to train nursing staff who would then serve as resources for other staff members. The program, which included inhouse and outside expert lecturers, addressed key pain management issues, such as the assessment process and the four components of pain (physical, psychological, social, and spiritual). For example, concerning assess-

ment the pain history is stressed as being critical to effective pain management. Consequently, components of a pain history should include the following:

- Significant previous and/or ongoing pain and effect on the patient;

- Previously used pain control methods found helpful or unhelpful;

- Patients' attitudes toward medications, including substance use/abuse;

- Typical coping responses for stress or pain;

- Psychological symptoms, such as depression, anxiety, or psychosis;

- Family expectations and beliefs concerning pain;

- Ways in which the patient describes or shows pain; and

- Patients' knowledge and expectations regarding pain management methods and receiving information about pain management.

The biggest educational component was the development of an in-service module on effective pain management. The module addresses the scope of the problem, barriers to effective pain management, and definitions. After reviewing the materials, staff are expected to be able to

- discuss the need to systematically assess patients' pain;

- identify key reasons for the undertreatment of pain;

- recognize the difference between acute, chronic, and cancer pain; and

- understand that assessment and treatment of pain is an ethical obligation of health care providers.

Pain Assessment and Management

The module, which includes a posttest, is available for in-service education for all staff.

In addition, mandatory in-services regarding the assessment and treatment of pain were presented to all staff. These in-services, which were held over a period of a year, included lectures on such topics as "Managing the Drug Seeking Patient." Numerous current articles on pain were circulated bimonthly via in-service boards to the nursing units. Staff received in-service credit for reading the articles and completing a posttest. The in-services were held at various times to give all staff an opportunity to attend. In addition, they were videotaped to give staff an opportunity to view them at their convenience. CARITAS Health Services also offered a pain management fair to highlight a wide range of treatment options, stressing interdisciplinary care.

In addition to offering a variety of educational opportunities, the committee developed and/or revised documentation. For example, it developed and implemented a standardized pain assessment tool to be used on units at CARITAS Medical Center for initial assessment and ongoing monitoring of patients' pain. The tool lists various pain rating scales, including a numerical, descriptor, and faces scales. The tool is now included in patient charts. For children and adolescent patients, at CARITAS Peace Center a "Feelings Sheet" is used to help them recognize their feelings and emotional pain. In addition, a spiritual assessment form was developed. The form includes specific questions about pain to address the psychosocial impact of pain in addition to the physical characteristics.

The committee either developed or made available other educational tools, such as traveling in-service boards with articles, a resource list of clinicians who provide nonpharmacological treatments, and a resource list for clinicians that includes articles, books, slides, and videotapes.

The committee developed a policy and procedure for pain management for inclusion in the nursing patient management section. The policy states that health care providers are obligated to manage pain and relieve patient suffering as part of their professional commitment. Furthermore, the successful management of physical and emotional pain will depend on the assessment, identification, and determination of intervention. Additionally, the policy calls for patient education regarding an individualized treatment plan.

The procedure calls for patients who present with symptoms or complaints of emotional/physical pain to be evaluated using a psychosocial, spiritual, and physical pain assessment. Based on the patient's identified needs, a specific plan of treatment will be developed. Treatment goals for pain relief will be determined by the patient and treatment team. The patient will be informed and educated about pharmacologic therapies and nonpharmacologic interventions. The patient will be treated respectfully, treated with different modalities when indicated, and be given medications safely and accurately. Patients in the later stages of a terminal illness will be administered medication to keep them comfortable and allow them to die with dignity. Based on continuous clinical assessment, the clinician will make a referral for the appropriate treatment modality. Finally, consultation with the Pain Management Center can be used as needed. The policy was approved in January 1996 and last reviewed in September 1998. The center's policy and procedure is similar to the corporate policy and procedure. The major difference is the Peace Center's willingness to consider more nonpharmacological therapies, notes Gatewood.

Although the CARITAS Medical Center has developed and implemented performance improvement measures for postoperative care, similar measures have not yet been instituted at the Peace Center. With its mission completed, the committee disbanded in 1997 and has not been reconvened, in part because SCN Health System has joined with other Catholic health systems across the country to form the Catholic Health Initiatives. Gatewood anticipates that once the center is more settled under the new parent com-

pany, focus will return to the management of both types of pain physical and emotional and additional resources will be allotted to this worthwhile endeavor. Meanwhile, Gatewood and Meyer are convinced that the assessment tools, and policies and procedures as well as education and orientation processes that were put into place have an ongoing impact on the quality of patient care. "Current staff are more aware of the impact of both emotional and physical pain on the quality of our patients' lives," says Gatewood.

Ambulatory Care Case Study:
Pain Management Center of Paducah

Established initially as a private medical office in 1989, the Pain Management Center of Paducah in Kentucky has evolved over the years into an ambulatory center that manages subacute, chronic, and cancer pain. The Pain Management Center also includes a subsidiary, Physical Therapy and Psychology, which provides complementary physical therapy, rehabilitation services, and psychological services. Persons served include individuals with complaints of enduring pain who have not responded to previous appropriate medical or surgical treatment; were treated inappropriately; or are seeking treatment for the first time for pain that interferes with their physical, psychological, social, and/or vocational functioning.

The program's objectives are as follows:

- Reduce or eliminate pain;

- Improve functional status;

- Increase level of activity;

- Return to work;

- Reduce dependence on others for activities of daily living;

- Maximize independence in mobility;

- Reduce pain behavior;

- Reduce intake of medications with potential for dependency;

- Improve psychological status;

- Reduce unnecessary and redundant medical care;

- Reduce or optimize health care expenditures; and

- Optimize patient satisfaction.

The Center comprises 45 employees, including three anesthesiologists with subspecialty in pain management, a psychologist, two physical therapists, 16 nurses, five surgical technicians, and administrative personnel, and espouses a multidisciplinary team approach to pain management. Evidence of that approach is the interdisciplinary team that holds at least monthly conferences for each person receiving treatment in two out of the three components (medical, psychological, and functional management) of the pain program. (See Figure 9.7 for Suggested Algorithm for Comprehensive Evaluation and Management of Chronic Pain.)

The Center's policies and procedures were initially established in 1992 by an interdisciplinary team consisting of a physician, psychologist, physical therapist, and two nurses. The following year, policies and procedures were expanded to meet criteria for chronic pain programs. The final modification of policies and procedures, which occurred in 1999, meets criteria for rehabilitation and surgery center programs, as well. Policies and procedures are evaluated and updated annually by key personnel including the medical director, medical staff, clinical director, nursing administrator, director of human resources, and the administrator. After modifications are made, they are approved by the Quality Management and Improvement Committee and the Medical Staff Executive Committee.

The Pain Management Center's Medical Director, Laxmaiah Manchikanti, MD, believes that proper procedure management requires the establishment of policies and procedures that meet the criteria of relevant accrediting bodies, such as the Joint Commission. When developing such policies for the Center, the importance of pain assessment was stressed, he recalls.

Figure 9-7. Suggested Algorithm for Comprehensive Evaluation and Management of Chronic Pain

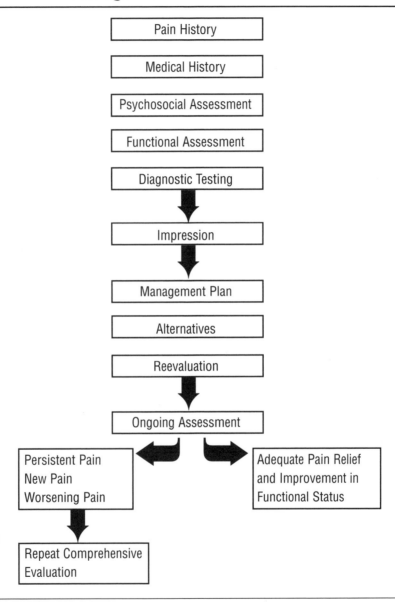

Source: The Pain Management Center of Paducah, Paducah, KY. Used with permission.

As part of pain management, all individuals seeking treatment are given an initial assessment that includes a physical and psychosocial status and health history. After an appointment is made, a comprehensive questionnaire is mailed to the persons seeking care with a request to complete it prior to arriving for the initial assessment. The 15-page questionnaire includes a pain; past, family, and social; and medical history. During the initial assessment, the individual served may be assessed for nutritional or functional status, and may undergo diagnostic testing. Persons served are reassessed and reevaluated at follow up visits, which can occur anywhere from two weeks to two years based on responsiveness to the treatment.

Pain assessment instruments used include the short form of McGill's Pain Questionnaire, a numerical pain rating scale, and a pain diagram. In addition, a patient questionnaire addresses modifying factors for pain and sleep disturbances as well as social and environmental influences.

Policies and procedures also address patient/family education, which is an essential component of Paducah's program. In fact, patient/family education begins prior to the initial assessment when individuals served are sent appropriate literature on various pain problems along with a brochure on patients' rights and responsibilities. Written materials focus on issues such as low back pain, neck pain, headaches, shingles, pain management, and physical therapy/psychology.

As part of the Pain Management Center's orientation of the patient and when appropriate, the family, policy and procedure is stated as follows:

- Communications are in a form (language, literacy level) which is easily understood by the person being served, the family, and/or the personal representative.

- The process of development of treatment is discussed with the person and, if appropriate, the family. There is a full discussion of how the person is to participate in goal setting and program planning, unless contraindicated by circumstances unique to the person.

- The programs and services are explained and discussed with the person, and if appropriate, the family.

- The mechanism by which the person's program will be managed is explained at or shortly after entrance/admission.

Providers also discuss the various sources of chronic pain and how it impacts every day life with individuals served during office visits. They provide literature in the form of pamphlets, handouts, and other sources of information or where to obtain such information (local arthritis support groups). Additionally, videotapes reviewing interventions, such as morphine pumps and spinal cord stimulators, are available.

As nursing documentation had to be modified to reflect the more multidisciplinary approach to pain management as the Center evolved, the aforementioned team reconvened to make those changes. The modifications, which took approximately six months to complete, primarily focused on procedural changes, such as pre- and post-op assessment.

After these changes were made, staff were apprised of them through a variety of educational interventions. For example, staff was required to attend in-service sessions, providers were sent to various relevant conferences, and continuing education courses were provided for nurses, physical therapists, and psychologists.

To date, a staff in-service session addressing a pain management topic is held every other month. Topics addressed include evaluation and management services, appropriate documentation, procedural assistance, patient follow up, as well as recognition and diagnosis of complications and appropriate interventions. Deleterious effects of uncontrolled pain, and myths regarding the use of invasive technology versus non-invasive methods to assess and manage pain are other common subjects. Sometimes, external speakers, such as practice management consultants, are brought in. In addition, pain management issues are addressed as part of new clinical staff orientation.

Approximately one year ago, using a combination of evidence and consensus the Center's interdisciplinary team developed and implemented clinical practice guidelines that address the use of interventional pain techniques in the management of chronic pain. The population covered includes all patients eligible for neural blockade suffering with chronic pain of either spinal or nonspinal origin. Manchikanti says the purpose of instituting these guidelines are to improve quality of care, patient outcomes, appropriateness of care, and efficiency and effectiveness; to increase patient access; and to achieve cost containment with demonstration of past benefit ratio. Although it plans to continue data collection for two years before analyzing the data, the Pain Management Center says there are already positive changes to patient care. For example, prior to guideline implementation, many patients received epidural injections as the first line of treatment. Now, the majority of patients receive facet blocks, which is a more appropriate use of these pain interventions.

The Pain Management Center plans to distribute these guidelines to other pain management centers nationwide as well as other organizations including Medicare, Medicaid, and third party payers. He is doing this through the auspices of the Association of Pain Management Anesthesiologists, a group of more than 300 pain specialists that he co-founded in 1998.

As part of its quality improvement efforts, the Pain Management Center collects data to measure functional outcomes, medical outcomes, disposition at discharge, status of postdischarge functional abilities, appropriate use of medication, effective management of pain, and cost-

effective treatment. Data are collected by three means: random chart analysis, a patient satisfaction questionnaire distributed to individuals served after each visit, and an annual patient opinion survey. When the charts are pulled, the person's status is compared at baseline, three months, six months, and one and two years. (See Figure 9.8 a-d for Comparison of Treatment Improvement Over Time.) The one-page survey developed in-house asks patients about their pain and functional status as well as physical and mental health. For example, if the individual's goal was to return to work and that occurred, then the functional status would be rated a "10" on a scale of 1 to 10. If the person's depression and anxiety is stable and he or she is on a low dose of medication, the scale would be rated a "5." The annual patient survey, which is mailed at year's end to all of the patients listed in the Center's directory, was designed to elicit patients' overall impression of the Center and the likelihood that they would recommend it to others. (See Figure 9.9 for General Aspects of 1998 Patient Opinion Survey.) The annual survey evaluations can even be used to compare the Center's performance from one year to the next. (See Figure 9.10 for Comparison of Favorable Opinion on General Aspects of Years 1997 and 1998.)

A statistician analyzes these data and presents them to the various providers at monthly staff meetings as well as to management at quarterly Quality Management and Improvement meetings. Further requirements in technology, cost savings, and improvement in outcome measures are incorporated. For example, the data revealed that no follow-up mechanism existed for missed appointments. Consequently, a chart would simply indicate that the individual served missed the appointment. A system involving the use of telephone calls and letters was established to follow

Figure 9.8 Comparison of Treatment Improvement Over Time

a. Three Month Post Treatment Improvement
Number of Patient = 69

	No Change	Mild Improvement	Moderate Improvement	Significant Improvement
1. Functional Status	4%	26%	22%	58%
2. Emotional adjustment & Coping skills	7%	33%	4%	55%
3. Maintain a productive Role	4%	22%	61%	13%
4. Reduce health care utilization	6%	16%	3%	75%
Average	5%	24%	23%	48%

b. Six Month Post Treatment Improvement
Number of Patient = 66

	No Change	Mild Improvement	Moderate Improvement	Significant Improvement
1. Functional Status	3%	23%	24%	50%
2. Emotional adjustment & Coping skills	5%	28%	8%	60%
3. Maintain a productive Role	3%	14%	65%	15%
4. Reduce health care utilization	6%	17%	0%	77%
Average	5%	20%	24%	51%

c. One Year Post Treatment Improvement
Number of Patient = 29

	No Change	Mild Improvement	Moderate Improvement	Significant Improvement
1. Functional Status	10%	31%	28%	31%
2. Emotional adjustment & Coping skills	11%	38%	11%	41%
3. Maintain a productive Role	7%	38%	48%	7%
4. Reduce health care utilization	11%	25%	0%	64%
Average	20%	32%	22%	36%

d. Overall Improvement

	3 Months	6 Months	12 Months	Average
1. Functional Status	96%	97%	90%	94%
2. Emotional adjustment & Coping skills	93%	95%	89%	92%
3. Maintain a productive Role	96%	97%	93%	95%
4. Reduce health care utilization	94%	94%	89%	92%
Average	95%	96%	90%	

Source: The Pain Management Center of Paducah, Paducah, KY. Used with permission.

Figure 9-9. General Aspects

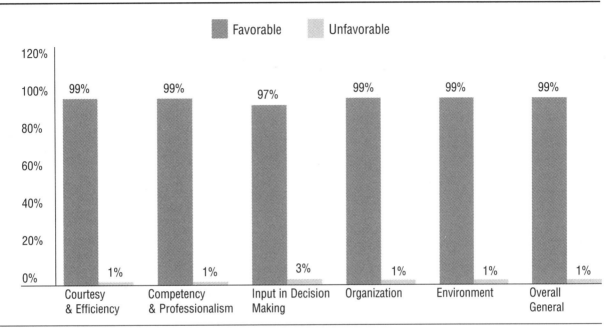

Source: The Pain Management Center of Paducah, Paducah, KY. Used with permission.

Figure 9-10. Comparison of Favorable Opinion on General Aspects of Years 1997 & 1998

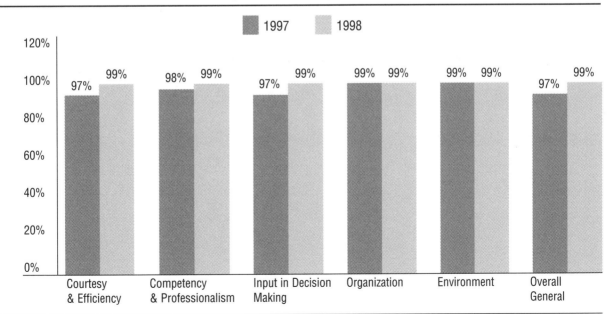

Source: The Pain Management Center of Paducah, Paducah, KY. Used with permission.

up all missed appointments until a resolution is made, thus ensuring that follow up is performed for all patients.

The Pain Management Center maintains that the goals of a pain management practice should be defined and reevaluated on a regular basis, ideally annually, using the principles of the "SWOT" (strengths, weaknesses, opportunities, and threats) analysis to do so.

"Physicians should realize that creating a pain management practice is dramatically different from operating room-based anesthesia or other types of medical or surgical practices," Manchikanti says. "Building a successful pain management practice takes time and hard work, but it is attainable by any competent physician who is willing to plan for success." He concludes, "It serves well to always remember the saying, 'Failing to plan is planning to fail.'"

REFERENCES AND READINGS

1. American Pain Society, American Academy of Pain Medicine, Janssen Pharmaceutical: Chronic pain in America: Roadblocks to relief. Study conducted by Roper Starch Worldwide, 1999.

2. Wolfe J, et al. Symptoms and suffering at the end of life in children with cancer. *New England Journal of Medicine* 342(5):326–333, Feb 2000.

3. Won A, et al. Correlates and management of nonmalignant pain in the nursing home. *Journal of the American Geriatrics Society* 47:936–942, 1999.

4. Desbiens NA, et al. Pain and satisfaction with pain control in seriously ill hospitalized adults: Findings from the SUPPORT research investigations. Critical Care Medicine 24(12):1953–1961, 1996.

5. Donovan M, Dillon P, McGuire L. Incidence and characteristics of pain in a sample of medical-surgical inpatients. *Pain* 56:69–87, Jul 1987.

6. Institue of Medicine. *Approaching Death: Improving Care at the End of Life.* Washington, DC: National Academy Press, 1997, p 5.

7. Lamberg, L. New guidelines on managing chronic pain in older persons. *Journal of the American Medical Association* 280(4):311, 1998.

8. Ferrell BA, Ferrell BR, Osterweil D. Pain in the nursing home. *Journal of the American Geriatric Society* 38(4):409–414, 1990.

9. Bernabei R, et al. Management of pain in elderly patients with cancer. *Journal of the American Medical Association* 279(23):1877–1882, Jun 17, 1998.

10. A controlled trial to improve care for seriously ill hospitalized patients; the study to understand prognoses and preferences for outcomes and risk for treatments (SUPPORT). The SUPPORT principal investigators, *Journal of the American Medical Association* 274(20):1591–1598, Nov 1995.

11. Brunier G, Carson MG, Harrison DE. What do nurses know and believe about patients with pain? Results of a hospital survey. *Journal of Pain and Symptom Management* 10(6):436–445, Aug 1995.

12. Ferrell BR, McGuire DB, Donovan MI. Knowledge and beliefs regarding pain in a sample of nursing faculty. *Journal of Professional Nursing* 9(2):79–88, Mar/Apr 1993.

13. Gibbs G. Nurses in private nursing homes: A study of their knowledge and attitudes to pain management in palliative care. *Palliative Medicine* 9(3):245–253, Jul 1995.

14. McCaffrey M, Thorpe D. Differences in perception of pain and the development of adversarial relationships among health care providers. In Hill CS & Fields WS (eds): Advances in Pain Research and Therapy, Volume 11. Drug Treatment of Cancer Pain in a Drug-Oriented Society. New York: Raven Press, 1989, 113–122.

15. Levin ML, Berry JI, Leiter J. Management of pain in terminally ill patients; physician reports of knowledge, attitudes, and behavior. *Journal of Pain and Symptom Management* 15(1):27–39, Jan 1998.

16. Drayer RA, Henderson J, Reidenberg M. Barriers to better pain control in hospitalized patients. *Journal of Pain and Symptom Management* 17(6):434–440, Jun 1999.

17. Cleeland CS. Undertreatment of cancer pain in elderly patients. *Journal of the American Medical Association* 279(23):1914–1915, Jun 17, 1998.

18. Breitbart W, Rosenfeld B, Passik SD. The Network Project: A multidisciplinary cancer education and training program in pain management, rehabilitation, and psychosocial issues. *Journal of Pain and Symptom Management* 15(1):18–26, Jan 1998.

19. Sloan PA, et al. Cancer pain education among family physicians. *Journal of Pain and Symptom Management* 14(2):74–81, Aug 1997.

20. Miller EH, et al. Institutionwide pain management improvement through the use of evidence-based content, strategies, resources, and outcomes. *Quality Management in Health Care* 7(2):28–40, Winter 1999.

21. McCaffery M, et al. Nurses' knowledge of opioid analgesic drugs and psychological dependence. *Cancer Nursing* 13(1):21–27, Feb 1990.

22. Von Roenn JH, et al. Physician attitudes and practice in cancer pain management. A survey from the Eastern Cooperative Oncology Group. *Ann Internal Medicine* 119(2):121–126, Jul 1993.

23. Vortherms R, Ryan P, Ward S: Knowledge of, attitudes toward, and barriers to pharmacologic management of cancer pain in a statewide random sample of nurses. *Research in Nursing and Health* 15(6):459–466, Dec 1992.

24. The management of chronic pain in older persons: AGS Panel on Chronic Pain in Older Persons. *Journal of the American Geriatric Society* 46(5):635–651, May 1998.

25. Model guidelines for the use of controlled substances for the treatment of pain. *Federation Bulletin* 85(2):84–87, 1998.

26. The Use of Opioids for the Treatment of Chronic Pain. A consensus statement from the American Academy of Pain Medicine and the American Pain Society. www.painmed.org.

27. Pasero C, et al. Chapter 16: Building institutional commitment to improving pain management. In McCaffery M: *Pain Clinical Manual.* St Louis, MO: Mosby, 1999.

28. Gordon DB, Dahl JL, Stevenson KK: *Building an Institutional Commitment to Pain Management: The Wisconsin Resource Manual for Improvement.* Madison, WI: Wisconsin Cancer Pain Initiative, 1997.

29. Weissman DE. Cancer pain education for physicians in practice: Establishing a new paradigm. *Journal of Pain and Symptom Management* 12(6):364–371, Dec 1996.

30. Heye ML, Goddard L. Teaching pain management: How to make it work. *Journal for Nurses in Staff Development* 15(1):27–36, Jan/Feb 1999.

31. Check all knowledge and attitude bases to get ready for pain management. *Joint Commission Benchmark* 1(2):1–3, Apr 1999.

32. Bookbinder M, et al. Implementing national standards for cancer pain management: Program model and evaluation. *Journal of Pain and Symptom Management* 12(6):334–347, Dec 1996.

33. Angelucci D, Quinn L, Handlin D. A pain management relief plan. *Nursing Management* 29(10):49–54, Oct 1998.

34. Tavris DR, et al. Evaluation of a local cooperative project to improve postoperative pain management in Wisconsin hospitals. *Quality Management in Health Care* 7(2):20–27, Winter 1999.

35. Jacox A, Carr DB, Payne R. New clinical-practice guidelines for the management of pain in patients with cancer. *New England Journal of Medicine* 330(9):651–655, Mar 3, 1994.

36. Lehna C, Seck L, Churches S. Development of an outcome measure to document pain relief for home hospice patients: A collaboration between nursing education and prac-tice. *American Journal of Hospice & Palliative Care* 15(6):343–351, Nov/Dec 1998.

37. Fins JJ. Public attitudes about pain and anal-gesics: Clinical implications. *Journal of Pain and Symptom Management* 13(3):169–171, Mar 1997.

38. Ward SE, et al. Patient-related barriers to management of cancer pain. Pain 52(3):319–324, Mar 1993.

39. Monti DA, Kunkel EJ. Management of chronic pain among elderly patients. *Psychiatric Services* 49(12):1537–1539, Dec 1998.

40. Gauthier JC, Finley GA, McGrath PJ. Children's self-report of postoperative pain intensity and treatment threshold: Determining the adequacy of medication. *Clinical Journal of Pain* 14(2):116–120, Jun 1998.

41. Palermo TM, Drotar DD, Lambert S. Psychosocial predictors of children's post-operative pain. *Clinical Nursing Research* 7(3):275–291, Aug 1998.

42. Fuller BF, et al. Testing a model of the nurs-ing assessment of infant pain. *Clinical Nursing Research* 8(1):69–83, Feb 1999.

43. Buchholz M, et al. Pain scores in infants: A modified infant pain scale versus visual ana-logue. *Journal of Pain and Symptom Management* 15(2):117–124, Feb 1998.

44. Breitbart W, et al. Patient-related barriers to pain management in ambulatory AIDS patients. *Pain* 76(1–2):9–16, May 1998.

45. Stephenson J. Experts say AIDS pain 'dramatically undertreated.' *Journal of the American Medical Asssociation* 276(17):1369–1370, Nov 6, 1996.

46. Quality Care at the End of Life: A consensus statement from the American Academy of Pain Medicine and the American Pain Society, 1998. www.painmed.org.

47. Briggs M, Dean KL. A qualitative analysis of the nursing documentation of post-operative pain management. *Journal of Clinical Nursing* 7(2):155–163, Mar 1998.

48. Dalton JA, et al. Changing the relationship among nurses' knowledge, self-reported behavior, and documented behavior in pain management: Does education make a difference? *Journal of Pain and Symptom Management* 12(5):308–319, Nov 1996.

49. Weber M, Huber C. Documentation of severe pain, opioid doses, and opioid-related side effects in outpatients with cancer: A retrospective study. *Journal of Pain and Symptom Management* 17(1): 49–54, Jan 1999.

50. Jadlos MA, et al. A pain management documentation tool. *Oncology Nursing Forum* 23(9):1451–1453, 1996.

51. Trowbridge R, et al. Determining the effectiveness of a clinical-practice intervention in improving the control of pain in outpatients with cancer. *Academic Medicine* 72(9):798–800, Sep 1997.

52. Janjan NA, et al. Teaching cancer pain management: Durability of educational effects of a role model program. *Cancer* 77(5):996–1001, Mar 1, 1996.

53. Daroszewski EB, Meehan DA: Pain, role play, and videotape: Pain management staff development in a community hospital. *Journal of Nursing Staff Development* 13(3):119-124, May/Jun 1997.

54. Wallace KG, et al. Lessons learned in implementing a staff education program in pain management in the acute care setting. *Journal of Nursing Staff Development* 13(1):24–31, Jan/Feb 1997.

55. Rischer JB, Childress SB. Cancer pain management: Pilot implementation of the AHCPR guideline in Utah. *Joint Commission Journal of Quality Improvement* 22(10):683–697, Oct 1996.

56. Griffie J, Weissman DE. Palliative medicine nurse preceptorship at the Medical College of Wisconsin. *Journal of Pain and Symptom Management* 12(6):360–363, Dec 1996.

57. Henley NS, et al. Replication of clinical innovations in multiple medical practices. *Joint Commission Journal of Quality Improvement* 24(11):623–639, Nov 1998.

58. Barnason S, et al. Utilizing an outcomes approach to improve pain management by nurses: A pilot study. *Clinical Nurse Specialist* 12(1):28–36, Jan 1998.

59. Starck PL, et al. Development of a pain management report card for an acute care setting. *Advanced Practice Nursing Quarterly* 3(2):57–63, Fall 1997.

60. Dalton JA, et al. Pain management issues: The cost of medications in rural settings. *Hospice Journal* 13(4):19–32, 1998.

61. McCaffery M, Ferrell BR. Nurses' knowledge of pain assessment and management: How much progress have we made? *Journal of Pain and Symptom Management* 14(3):175–188, Sep 1997.

62. Benjamin LJ, et al. *Guideline for the Management of Acute and Chronic Pain in Sickle-Cell Disease.* Glenview, IL: American Pain Society, 1999.

63. American Pain Society. *Principles of Analgesic Use in the Treatment of Acute Pain and Cancer Pain.* 4th ed. Glenview, IL: American Pain Society, 1998.

64. Acute Pain Management Guideline Panel. Acute Pain Management: Operative or Medical Procedures and Trauma: *Clinical Practice Guideline No. 1.* AHCPR Publication No. 92-0032. Rockville, MD: Agency for Health Care Policy and Research, Feb 1992.

65. Jacox A, et al. Management of Cancer Pain. *Clinical Practice Guideline No. 9.* AHCPR Publication No. 94-0592. Rockville, MD: Agency for Health Care Policy and Research, Mar 1994.

66. Practice guidelines for chronic pain management: A report by the American Society of Anesthesiologists Task Force on Pain Management, Chronic Pain Section. *Anesthesiology* 86(4):995-1004, Apr 1997.

67. Acupuncture: NIH Consensus Statement. 15(5):1–34, Nov 3-5, 1997.

68. Donovan M, Laack KD. Individually reported effectiveness of therapy for chronic pain. *Clinical Nursing Research* 7(4):423–439, Nov 1998.

69. Bostrom M. Summary of the Mayday Fund Survey: Public attitudes about pain and analgesics. *Journal of Pain and Symptom Management* 13:166–171, Mar 1997.

70. Wells N, Johnson RL, Wujcik D. Development of a short version of the Barriers Questionnaire. *Journal of Pain and Symptom Management* 15(5):294–298, May 1998.

71. Paice JA, Toy C, Shott S. Barriers to cancer pain relief: Fear of tolerance and addiciton. *Journal of Pain and Symptom Management* 16(1):1–9, Jul 1998.

72. Ferrell BR, Rhiner M, Ferrell BA. Development and implementation of a pain education program. *Cancer Suppl* 72(11):3426–3432, Dec 1, 1993.

73. deWit R, et al. A pain education program for chronic cancer pain patients: Follow-up results from a randomized controlled trial. *Pain* 73(1):55–69, Oct 1997.

Additional Readings

Borromeo AR, Windle PE. Benchmarking for unrelieved pain in a postanesthesia care unit. *Best Practices in Benchmarking in Healthcare* 2(1):20–23, Jan/Feb 1997.

Boyer BA. SPARKS are flying in Philadelphia. *Hospital & Healthcare News,* Jan/Feb 1999.

A clinical model for procedural pain interventions: Practice guidelines for comprehensive and individualized application. *Families, Systems & Health* 16(1/2):103–126, Spring/Summer 1998.

Foreman MD, Wykle M. Nursing standard-of-practice protocol: Sleep disturbances in elderly patients. *Geriatric Nursing* 16(5):238–243, Sept/Oct 1995.

Fulmer TT, Mion LF, Bottrell MM, NICHE faculty. Pain management protocol. *Geriatric Nursing* 17(5):222–226, Sep/Oct 1996.

Gallagher RM. Outcomes and moral hazards in the medical culture of opiod phobia. *Clinical Journal of Pain* 14(3):185–186, Sept 1998.

Grond S, et al. Validation of World Health Organization guidelines for cancer pain relief during the last days and hours of life. *Journal of Pain and Symptom Management* 6(7): 411–422, Oct 1991.

Joranson DE, Gilson AM. Improving pain management through policy making and education for medical regulators. *Journal of Law, Medicine & Ethics* 24(4): 344–347, Winter 1996.

Martino AM. In search of a new ethic for treating patients with chronic pain: What can medical boards do? *Journal of Law, Medicine & Ethics* 26(4): 332–349, Winter 1998.

Petersen C: Current healthcare delivery system thwarts pain management. *Managed Healthcare* 8(9)38–40, Sep 1998.

Portenoy RK. Opioid therapy for chronic nonmalignant pain: A review of the critical issues. *Journal of Pain and Symptom Management* 11(4): 203–217, Apr 1996.

Ward S, Donovan M, Max MB. A survey of the nature and perceived impact of quality improvement activities in pain management. *Journal of Pain and Symptom Management* 15(6): 365–373, Jun 1998.

Appendix A:

RESOURCES

Preceptorships, Observerships, Fellowships

Beth Israel Hospital
Kathy Horvath
330 Brookline Ave.
Boston, MA 02215
617/667-8000
Preceptorship is arranged on individual request; acute, chronic nonmalignant, and/or cancer pain content tailored to meet participants' needs; nurses, pharmacists, and physicians may attend.

Fox Chase Cancer Center
Karen Davis
7701 Burholme Ave.
Philadelphia, PA 19111
215/728-3009
Preceptorship is arranged on individual request; cancer pain content tailored to meet participants' needs; time is spent with the entire health care team in both the inpatient and outpatient settings; nurses, pharmacists, and physicians may attend.

Mayo St. Luke's Hospital
Anesthesia Department and Training
and Education Department
4201 Belfort Rd.
Jacksonville, FL 32224
904/296-3712 or 904/953-8807
Prepares attending nurses to be PRNs in their own institutions.

Mercy Hospital Medical Center
Pain Management Services
400 University Ave.
Des Moines, IA 50314-1101
515/247-3172 or 515/247-3239
Comprehensive program focusing on acute, chronic nonmalignant, and cancer pain; targeted for nurses, but pharmacists and physicians also may attend.

Network Project
Memorial Sloan-Kettering Cancer Center
Department of Pain and Palliative Care
1275 York Ave.
New York, NY 10021
Send written request to attend to address above. Two-week observership in cancer pain management, psychosocial oncology, and cancer rehabilitation for health care professions from any discipline. Participants are selected on the basis of their potential to educate and train others within their own institution and community.

Pain Assessment and Management

Nurse Fellowship in Pain and Palliative Care

Memorial Sloan-Kettering Cancer Center
Department of Pain and Palliative Care
1275 York Ave.
New York, NY 10021

Send written request to attend to address above. One-year internship in cancer pain management and palliative care for masters prepared nurses.

Palliative Care Nurse Preceptorship Program

Medical College of Wisconsin
9200 W. Wisconsin Ave.
Milwaukee, WI 53226
414/257-6117

A three-day clinical and didactic program that focuses on pain and symptom management at end of life.

Pain Resource Nurse Programs

Dr. Betty Ferrell
City of Hope National Medical Center
1500 East Duarte Rd.
Duarte, CA 91010-3012
626/301-8346

Teaches attending nurses how to develop a PRN program in their own institutions. City of Hope also offers a pain education program for selected clinical nurse specialists and quality assurance/improvement coordinators.

Source: American Pain Society (www.ampainsoc.org)

Resources for Pain Professionals

The American Academy of Pain Medicine
4700 W. Lake Ave.
Glenview, IL 60025
847/375-4731
Fax 847/375-6331
www.painmed.org

American Academy of Pediatrics
141 Northwest Point Boulevard
Elk Grove Village, IL 60007-1098
847/434-4000
847/434-8000
www.aap.org

American Headache Society
19 Mantua Road
Mount Royal, NJ 08061
856/423-0043
Fax 856/423-0082
www.ahsnet.org

The American Pain Society
4700 W. Lake Ave.
Glenview, IL 60025
847/375-4715
Fax 847/375-6315
www.ampainsoc.org

American Society of Addiction Medicine
4601 North Park Ave, Arcade Suite 101
Chevy Chase, MD 20815
301/656-3920
Fax 301/656-3815
www.asam.org

American Society of Anesthesiologists
520 N. Northwest Highway
Park Ridge, IL 60068-2573
847/825-5586
Fax 847/825-1692
www.asahq.org

American Society of Pain Management Nurses
7794 Grow Drive
Pensacola, FL 32514
888/34-ASPMN (342-7766)
Fax 850/484-8762
www.aspmn.org

American Society of Regional Anesthesia
P.O. Box 11086
Richmond, VA 23230-1086
804/282-0010
Fax 804/282-0090
www.asra.com

International Association for the Study of Pain®
909 NE 43rd St., Suite 306
Seattle, WA 98105-6020
206/547-6409
Fax 206/547-1703
www.halcyon.com/iasp

The National Guideline Clearinghouse
6010 Executive Boulevard, Suite 300
Rockville, MD 20852
www.guideline.gov

Source: American Pain Society (www.ampainsoc.org)

Resources for Persons with Pain

American Chronic Pain Association

Has over 800 peer support group chapters
worldwide; various written materials available; no
physician/counseling referrals.
P.O. Box 850
Rocklin, CA 95677
916/632-0922
Fax 916/632-3208
www.theacpa.org

American Foundation for Urologic Disease

Prostate Cancer Support Network
Has written material; access to about 400 national
support groups; no physician referrals.
300 West Pratt St, Suite 40
Baltimore, MD 21201
410/727-2908 or 800/828-7866
www.afud.org

American Pain Foundation

A consumer information, education and advocacy
organization dedicated to helping people in pain.
The American Pain Foundation Website is an
online resource center for people with pain, their
families, friends, caregivers, the media,
legislators, and the general public.
111 S. Calvert Street, Suite 2700
Baltimore, MD 21202
410/385-5276
Fax 410/385-1832
www.painfoundation.org

The American Pain Society (APS)

The American Pain Society (APS) is a multi-
disiplinary organization of basic and clinical
scientists, practicing clinicians, policy analysts,
and others.
4700 W. Lake Avenue
Glenview, IL 60025
847/375-4715
Fax 847/375-6315
www.ampainsoc.org

Arthritis Foundation

Has written material; support groups; will provide list of arthritis specialists in patient's area.
1330 W. Peachtree
Atlanta, GA 30309
404/872-7100 or 800/283-7800
www.arthritis.org

Candlelighters Childhood Cancer Foundation

Has written materials; over 400 peer support
groups and contacts for all family members
nationwide.
8323 SW Freeway, Suite 435
Houston, TX 77074
713/270-4700
Fax 713/270-9802
www.candle.org

Cancer Care, Inc
Has written material; telephone support groups
and counseling; will locate other community services in patient area.
275 7th Avenue
New York, NY 10001
212/302-2400 or 800/813-4673
Fax 212/719-0263
www.cancercareinc.org

Appendix B:

CONSENSUS STATEMENTS ON THE USE OF OPIOIDS

The use of opioids for the treatment of chronic pain: A consensus statement from the American Academy of Pain Medicine and American Pain Society

Source: *Clinical Journal of Pain* 1997 Mar;13(1):6-8

I. The management of pain is becoming a higher priority in the United States. In the last several years, health policymakers, health professionals, regulators, and the public have become increasingly interested in the provision of better pain therapies. This is evidenced, in part, by the U.S. Department of Health and Human Services' dissemination of Clinical Practice Guidelines for the management of acute pain and cancer pain. These publications, which have been endorsed by AAPM and APS, state that opioids, sometimes called "narcotic analgesics," are an essential part of a pain management plan. There is currently no nationally accepted consensus for the treatment of chronic pain not due to cancer, yet the economic and social costs of chronic pain are substantial, with estimates ranging in the tens of billions of dollars annually.

II. Current conditions dictate the need for a joint consensus statement of two major national pain organizations. AAPM and APS believe that the United States is in a critical phase of state-level policy development with respect to the use of opioids in pain treatment. In this regard, there has been recent activity in state legislatures (such as intractable pain treatment acts and the establishment of pain commissions) and at the regulatory level (statements of policy from state boards of medical examiners). In response to inquiries from concerned boards, AAPM and APS wish to encourage a dialogue with regulators about the appropriate relation between law and the practice of pain medicine. The purpose of laws that govern controlled substances and professional conduct is to protect the public. Our objective is for state policies to recognize but not interfere with the medical use of opioids for pain relief, while continuing to address the issue of prescribing that may contribute to drug abuse and diversion. It is imperative that this statement not be misconstrued as advocating the imprudent use of opioids. Rather, if a practitioner decides to treat chronic pain with opioids, this document should serve as a guide for both the practitioner and regulators with regard to the judicious use of these drugs in the course of medical practice.

III. Pain is often managed inadequately, despite the ready availability of safe and effective treatments. Many strategies and options exist to treat chronic noncancer pain. Since chronic pain is not a single entity but may have myriad causes and perpetuating factors, these strategies and options vary from behavioral methods and rehabilitation approaches to the use of a number of different medications, including opioids.

Pain is one of the most common reasons people consult a physician, yet it frequently is inadequately treated, leading to enormous social cost in the form of lost productivity, needless suffering, and excessive healthcare expenditures.

Impediments to the use of opioids include concerns about addiction, respiratory depression and other side effects, tolerance, diversion, and fear of regulatory action.

IV. Current information and experience suggest that many commonly held assumptions need modification.

Addiction: Misunderstanding of addiction and mislabeling of patients as addicts result in unnecessary withholding of opioid medications. Addiction is a compulsive disorder in which an individual becomes preoccupied with obtaining and using a substance, the continued use of which results in a decreased quality of life. Studies indicate that the de novo development of addiction when opioids are used for the relief of pain is low. Furthermore, experience has shown that known addicts can benefit from the carefully supervised, judicious use of opioids for the treat-

ment of pain due to cancer, surgery, or recurrent painful illnesses such as sickle cell disease.

Respiratory depression and other side effects: Fear of inducing respiratory depression is often cited as a factor that limits the use of opioids in pain management. It is now accepted by practitioners of the specialty of pain medicine that respiratory depression induced by opioids tends to be a short-lived phenomenon, generally occurs only in the opioid-naive patient, and is antagonized by pain. Therefore, withholding the appropriate use of opioids from a patient who is experiencing pain on the basis of respiratory concerns is unwarranted. Other side effects, such as constipation, can usually be managed by attention to diet, along with the regular use of stool softeners and laxatives. Sedation and nausea, possible early side effects, usually dissipate with continued use.

Tolerance: It was previously thought that the development of analgesic tolerance limited the ability to use opioids efficaciously on a long-term basis for pain management. Tolerance, or decreasing pain relief with the same dosage over time, has not proven to be a prevalent limitation to long-term opioid use. Experience with treating cancer pain has shown that what initially appears to be tolerance is usually progression of the disease. Furthermore, for most opioids, there does not appear to be an arbitrary upper dosage limit, as was previously thought.

Diversion: Diversion of controlled substances should be a concern of every health professional, but efforts to stop diversion should not interfere with prescribing opioids for pain management. Attention to patterns of prescription requests and the prescribing of opioids as part of an ongoing relationship between a patient and a health care provider can decrease the risk of diversion.

V. Policy is evolving. State law and policy about opioid use are currently undergoing revision. The trend is to adopt laws or guidelines that specifically recognize the use of opioids to treat intractable pain. These statements serve as indicators of increased public awareness of the sequelae of undertreated pain and help clarify that the use of opioids for the relief of chronic pain is a legitimate medical practice.

VI. Accepted principles of practice for the use of opioids should be promulgated. Due to concerns about regulatory scrutiny, physicians need guidance as to what principles should generally be followed when prescribing opioids for chronic or recurrent pain states. Regulators have also expressed a need for guidelines to help them to distinguish legitimate medical practice from questionable practice and to allow them to appropriately concentrate investigative, educational, and disciplinary efforts, while not interfering with legitimate medical care.

VII. Principles of good medical practice should guide the prescribing of opioids. AAPM and APS believe that guidelines for prescribing opioids should be an extension of the basic principles of good professional practice.

Evaluation of the patient: Evaluation should initially include a pain history and assessment of the impact of pain on the patient, a directed physical examination, a review of previous diagnostic studies, a review of previous interventions, a drug history, and an assessment of coexisting diseases or conditions.

Treatment plan: Treatment planning should be tailored to both the individual and the presenting problem. Consideration should be given to different treatment modalities, such as a formal pain rehabilitation program, the use of behavioral strategies, the use of noninvasive techniques, or the use of medications, depending upon the physical and psychosocial impairment related to the pain. If a trial of opioids is selected, the physician should ensure that the patient or the patient's guardian is informed of the risks and benefits of opioid use and the conditions under which opioids will be prescribed. Some practitioners find a written agreement specifying these conditions to be useful.

An opioid trial should not be done in the absence of a complete assessment of the pain complaint.

Consultation as needed: Consultation with a specialist in pain medicine or with a psychologist may be warranted, depending on the expertise of the practitioner and the complexity of the presenting problem. The management of pain inpatients with a history of addiction or a comorbid psychiatric disorder requires special consideration, but does not necessarily contraindicate the use of opioids.

Periodic review of treatment efficacy: Review of treatment efficacy should occur periodically to assess the functional status of the patient, continued analgesia, opioid side effects, quality of life, and indications of medication misuse. Periodic reexamination is warranted to assess the nature of the pain complaint and to ensure that opioid therapy is still indicated. Attention should be given to the possibility of a decrease in global function or quality of life as a result of opioid use.

Documentation: Documentation is essential for supporting the evaluation, the reason for opioid prescribing, the overall pain management treatment plan, any consultations received, and periodic review of the status of the patient.

VIII. The Mission Statements of AAPM and APS are consistent with this collaborative effort. The American Academy of Pain Medicine is the AMA-recognized specialty society of physicians who practice pain medicine. The American Pain Society is the national chapter of the International Association for the Study of Pain and is composed of physicians, nurses, psychologists, scientists, and members of other disciplines who have an interest in the study and treatment of pain.

The mission of the American Academy of Pain Medicine is to enhance pain medicine practice in this country by promoting a socioeconomic and political climate conducive to the effective and efficient practice of pain medicine and by ensuring quality medical care by physicians specializing in pain medicine, for patients in need of such services.

The mission of the American Pain Society is to serve people in pain by advancing research, education, treatment, and professional practice. The undertreatment of pain in today's society is not justified. This joint consensus statement has been produced pursuant to the missions of both organizations, to help foster a practice environment in which opioids may be used appropriately to reduce needless suffering from pain.

The statement was prepared by the following committee members:
J. David Haddox, DDS MD (Chair);
David Joranson, MSSW (Vice Chairman);
Robert T. Angarola, Esq.; Albert Brady, MD;
Daniel B. Carr, MD;
E. Richard Blonsky, MD; Kim Burchiel, MD;
Melvin Gitlin, MD; Matthew Midcap, MD;
Richard Payne, MD; Dana Simon, MD;
Sridhar Vasudevan, MD; Peter Wilson, MBBS, PhD. Consultant, Russell K. Portenoy, MD.

Approved by the AAPM Board of Directors on June 29, 1996

Approved by the APS Executive Committee on August 20, 1996
American Academy of Pain Medicine
4700 W. Lake Avenue
Glenview, IL 60025-1485
847/375-4731
Fax 847/375-4777
E-mail: aapm@amctec.com
www.painmed.org

American Pain Society
4700 W. Lake Avenue
Glenview IL 60025-1485
847/375-4715
Fax: 847/375-4777
E-mail: info@ampainsoc.org
www.ampainsoc.org

INDEX